The Hell In Your Mind

By Carol A. Cobb

Daily Dominion Publishing
2937 Glen Darby Court
San Jose, California 95148

ISBN: 978-1-7350869-2-7

Printed in the USA

For more information visit

DailyDominion.com

Dedication

People may wonder what prompted me to write a book like this. It mostly came from my own experiences in dealing with mental and emotional issues. A lot of it has come from helping other people deal with theirs. I didn't go looking for problems in my life. They just showed up on my doorstep. A lot of these problems were things that had been brewing for a long time. It was just a combination of the right circumstances and timing that caused them to pop up to the surface. I could say the experience of getting free was like untangling a ball of string that was full of knots.

It is not the purpose of this book to tell my story in detail. Frankly, I would rather forget a lot of it and only keep what I have learned and profited from. If you are looking for lots of details and a play-by-play account of my battle with mental and emotional issues you won't find them here. I decided the reason to write this was to share what I have learned about getting free and getting healed. I have added a few examples of my own experiences to help illustrate the points made but that's all.

My experiences were very real. They had a dramatic impact on my life. Most of it was rooted in rejection thinking, insecurity and fear, and generational curses from occult and sexual sin. There was a lot of demonic oppression in the form of tormenting thoughts and pictures in my mind, oppressive dreams and nightmares, panic attacks, and struggling with the fear and the feeling that I was losing my mind. There were times I felt I was behind enemy lines finding out what it was like to live under the burden of mental and emotional struggles. God had a reason for it all.

This book is dedicated to all who have lived or are now living through hell because of mental and emotional problems. I want to share with you what I learned and what God showed me about how to untangle the knots without breaking the string. My experiences are not something I go broadcasting to everyone I meet. Not a lot of people know about my story. I mean, really, who wants everyone to know they have had mental problems? I am writing the book because I believe what I have learned can help others. I pray it will help those who read it to find wholeness, peace and restoration of their minds in the image of Christ.

Carol Cobb – May, 2020

Table of Contents

*"Stone walls do not a prison make,
nor iron bars a cage"*

Richard Lovelace – 1642

Introduction

Not too long ago I was putting a load of wash into the dryer. I stuffed all the wet clothes in, set the dial to the right cycle and pushed the start button. Later I came back to empty out the dryer and fold up the clothes. But when I opened it up and started to take them out, I found they were still pretty wet. I thought maybe someone had come and shut the machine off before it had a chance to complete the cycle so I set it again, started it again and went to take care of some other chores. When I came back the second time I found the clothes were still very damp. I couldn't figure out what was wrong until I pulled out the filter to check it. The dryer filter was loaded with lint and hardly any air was getting through. So I pulled all the lint out, put the filter back in and restarted the dryer a third time. This time, when I came back, the clothes were dry. As I started to take them out to fold them, the thought came to me that people's lives are a lot like the dryer (isn't it wonderful how God can show you things using the most boring tasks of life?). I thought about how so many people are not able to function very well and are not fulfilling their God-given assignments in life because the filters on their minds have not been taken out and cleaned. God's truth is not getting through all the "lint" and their lives are still being directed and controlled by wrong thinking.

I know my own life was. For many years things I thought and believed about God, myself, other people, and why my life was the way it was were wrong. I made choices and decisions based on my wrong thinking and then wondered why my life wasn't going anywhere and why I experienced constant frustration and disappointment. It wasn't till I believed in Jesus and was born again at the age of 19 that I began to discover how much of my belief system was composed of lies and deception. I had no idea then how much time and effort it was going to take to rid my mind of wrong thinking, ungodly mindsets, and demonic oppression and interference. It's probably just as well. If I had known I would have been too discouraged to start! Sometimes God only tells us as much as we need to know to get going.

Ripples in the water

Did you know your mind has a filter? When you experience life, those experiences are processed through the filter of your belief system. This belief system tells you what to think about what you experience. Why is this important? It is important because what you think will determine how you react. And your reactions and choices will bring consequences. It's called sowing and reaping. Your choices today determine where you end up tomorrow and the choices you make tomorrow determine where you go the day after that and so on. And your choices don't just affect you.

Picture in your mind what happens when you throw a rock into a pool of still water. Ripples begin to fan out from where the rock entered the water. Now picture five or six rocks being thrown into the water at the same time. As the ripples begin to radiate out from where the rocks hit the water they eventually begin to run into the ripples caused by the other rocks. They start to overlap and interfere with each other.

The choices we make every day have the same effect. You may not see how what you do today affects someone tomorrow but your choices will have consequences for others as well as for yourself. It is important to know that our choices are being motivated by right thinking.

The purpose of this book is to help you renew your mind. We will talk about how belief systems are formed and how beliefs affect behavior. We will talk about God's power to transform lives by transforming how we think. And we will talk about how to fill our minds with truth and to develop a kingdom-oriented mindset that is able to discern and come into agreement with the will of God.

It took time, after I came to Christ, for the Holy Spirit to point out where my beliefs were skewed, distorted, or just downright false. The process continues to this day. It took some time to change my thinking habits so I no longer allowed old patterns and beliefs to govern my life. It took time to identify and get rid of the demonic influences that had wormed their way into my mind and personality. During the process I had to let God show me what truthful, godly thinking was.

It took time to create new thinking habits and patterns. But eventually the fruit of a redeemed mind began to show up in my life. I would like to share what I have learned with you. These are not things I learned by reading books. These are things I learned because I put them into practice. Allow the Holy Spirit, as you read, to begin to target those things in your thinking and mindsets that he wants to change. You will never regret that you did.

The Need for a Renewed Mind

"Do not conform any longer to the pattern of this world, but be transformed by the renewing of your mind. Then you will be able to test and approve what God's will is – his good and pleasing and perfect will." (Romans 12: 2)

All of us who believe in Jesus want to know what his will is don't we? Why does it seem so hard for so many of us to find out what it is? Does he not want to tell us? Of course God wants us to know his will. We can't do it if we don't know what it is. The verse above offers a clue as to what might be the source of some of our difficulty in knowing God's will. In Romans 12:2 Paul directly relates the ability to know God's will with being transformed (changed) and no longer living according to the pattern of the world. And he says this transformation comes from having our minds renewed. To recognize and understand God's will you have to stop thinking and living the way the world does. To stop thinking and living the way the world does you have to have your mind renewed, or changed.

When you use a pattern to make a dress, every dress made from that pattern will look exactly alike. If you don't want to have that same dress anymore you need to find a different pattern to make your new dress with. If you don't want your life to look like it did before you became a follower of Jesus you need a new pattern to follow. If you keep using the same patterns that you did before you got saved, you shouldn't be surprised if your "dress" doesn't look any different than it did before. You can't create a "kingdom" life with a worldly pattern.

To "renew" means to make like new, to rebuild, to begin again. God wants to take our thinking and mindsets back to what they would have been if sin and the fall had never happened. In short, if you are still operating according to old, sinful, worldly mindsets and belief systems (patterns), there will be no change or transformation in your life and you will have a hard time discerning what God's will and purpose are. Or, if you have some idea of what his will is, you may have a hard time thinking of it as being good and pleasing and perfect. God's will is not going to look like something you want to do if you have an old, worldly, un-renewed mind.

As someone who has been in ministry for many years I have a lot of people come to me for prayer. Most of them want to pray that things in their life will change in some way. Many of them seem to be stuck in cycles of defeat and aimless wandering. Some want a quick fix. They want someone to pray, wave their hand over the spot, and make things different right now (usually, without any effort on their part). What they don't realize is change doesn't usually come that way. Even for church people. Yes, God can and will change circumstances quickly in answer to prayer. However, it is one thing to change circumstances; it's another thing entirely to change you. He is after a deeper, more permanent kind of change than just to make you feel better at the moment.

God's wants to change you so you will be able to recognize his love. And so you will recognize his will and do it. He wants us to be transformed so people can see a difference between those of us who love and serve God and those who do not. He wants to make us like Jesus so when people are around us they get a truthful representation of who God is and what he is like. In order for us to be able to live like Jesus we have learn to think like Jesus. This is what we call a kingdom mindset. A kingdom mindset is learning to think like Jesus, where you start to see things from his perspective and from the point of view of his eternal kingdom.

Perhaps you can remember when you were small and got stuck behind a crowd of people who were preventing you from seeing something you wanted to see. It might have been a parade or the animals at the zoo. Because everyone was bigger than you, you could not see past them.

But maybe your dad picked you up and put you up on his shoulders. All of a sudden you were as big as the other big people and could see everything they could see. The obstacles were gone. You could now see from the same point of view as your father because you were up high on the same level as he was.

The Bible tells us we have been raised up in Christ and seated with him in heavenly places (Ephesians 2:6). Our Father God wants to pick us up and carry us around on his shoulders so we can see things from the same perspective and point of view he does.

True transformation (change) can only come when a person's belief system changes. Until you begin to think differently and see things from a different point of view, any change will only be superficial and short-lived. You can see this principle at work every year in January as people make lists of resolutions about how they are going to change in the coming year.

Making a resolution to change has almost become a joke

because so few people ever stick with theirs long enough to really see any permanent change. Usually such resolutions start with great exertion of will power and good intentions. After a while though, the will power wears out and people slide right back into old habits. The problem for a lot of them is they are trying to change their behavior without changing their thinking.

For example, someone who is overweight might try really hard to diet and lose weight. But until they confront their beliefs and attitudes about food and the role it is to play in their lives they will usually fail to stick with the diet very long.

This is also why religion is hard. Religion is all about following rules and trying hard to be good. These rules are imposed from the outside and are supposed to work their way in and make the person change. It's hard to be good outside if inside you don't really want to be good.

Change, in God's economy, comes from the inside and works its way out. A person who is born again is changed on the inside and no longer wants to do what isn't right. Outward signs of change come because the person inside has changed; belief has changed and, with it, perspective has changed. It is only natural that choices and behavior will follow along.

Ungodly mindsets

All of us lived in ungodliness, sin, and with a worldly mindset (pattern of thinking), often for years and years before we became followers of Jesus. Our mindsets and belief systems were developed in a climate that was devoid of the knowledge of the truth, in a world system without the true knowledge of God:

"Furthermore, since they did not think it worthwhile to retain the knowledge of God, he gave them over to a depraved mind, to do what ought not to be done." (Romans 1: 28)

Sin results in a depraved mind that cannot recognize truth. As sinful people turned aside from the true knowledge of God, their minds became deceived and hardened to where they were not able to see the truth any longer. The entire world system we know today has been formed over generations as people have turned away from the true knowledge of God.

Ideas of what is "normal" and "right" develop from what we see and experience day by day as we live in the world. And what we see and experience every day before we are born again is a world formed by sin and wickedness. So sin and wickedness become "normal" to us because that is all we know. We must realize that worldly, sinful mindsets and beliefs are not "normal" for God's people. The Holy Spirit aims to re-acquaint us with normal and right as God determines them to be:

> "When the Counselor comes, whom I will send to you from the Father, the Spirit of truth who goes out from the Father, he will testify about me."
> (John 15: 26)

> "I have much more to say to you, more than you can now bear. Burt when he, the Spirit of truth, comes, he will guide you into all truth." (John 16: 12-13)

If you just automatically had your mind renewed when you received salvation there would be no need for a Counselor to lead you into truth. You need this Counselor because so much of what you have believed to be true and right isn't.

Only the Spirit of God can show you truth because he is the only one who knows what truth is. This is why he is called the Spirit of Truth. He is the only one who can show us where our thinking and beliefs have been influenced and shaped by the devil's lies and deception.

All the old programming of the world and from the devil must be cleaned out and your mind must be re-established in truth if you are to be conformed to the image of Christ and represent his kingdom to the world.

True freedom

Jesus said to know truth was to be free (John 8:32). From this statement we can deduct first, that truth exists, and second, that it is possible to know truth. Truth is registered in the mind. Compare this with what Jesus says about Satan. In John 8 he calls Satan the "father of lies". The devil is known throughout scripture as a liar and deceiver. His kingdom is founded on lies and deceit and that is how he operates - by means of lies and deception. So any mindset or belief system that is built or acquired as a result of living in agreement with the world (and by default, the kingdom of darkness) will also be based in lies and deception. It is impossible for it to be truthful because the devil cannot produce what he does not possess.

"Jesus said to them,

> "If God were your Father, you would love me, for I came from God and now am here. I have not come on my own; but he sent me. Why is my language not clear to you? Because you are

10

unable to hear what I say. (Remember how we said an ungodly mindset makes it hard to discern the will of God?) You belong to your father, the devil, and you want to carry out your father's desires. He was a murderer from the beginning, not holding to the truth, for there is no truth in him. When he lies, he speaks his native language, for he is a liar and the father of lies." (John 8: 42-44)

The devil cannot be truthful because there is no truth in him. Whatever he constructs will not produce or be in agreement with truth. In comparison, Jesus many times in the gospels uses the phrase, "I tell you the truth". He challenges accepted beliefs and contrasts them with truth. You can see this all through the Sermon on the Mount (Matthew 5, 6, 7) where Jesus says, "You have heard it said . . ." and "But I tell you . . .".

Truth and perception are not necessarily the same things. Truth exists even if nobody wants to believe it. God is the creator of the universe. This is truth. There are not a lot of people today who believe it. That doesn't stop it from being true. Perception is what is seen or perceived. Perception is altered depending on one's point of view, or attitude. My house is small. This is a perception. When I see a house that is much smaller than mine, my perception changes and now my house appears to be big in comparison.

New information and new experiences can alter perception. This is why Jesus did not say "what you see will make you free", or "what you feel will make you free". He knew perception is not stable unless it is grounded in something more permanent than what we happen to see or feel at the moment.

Truth does not change as perception can. New experiences

and changes of attitude do not alter truth. It remains the same. Our perceptions must have something to which they can be compared so we can tell if we are "seeing" correctly. What we have is the word of God, the Bible, and the indwelling presence of the Spirit of Truth. The knowledge of truth will affect your perception and is the only thing that will fix and stabilize it. Truth must determine your perception; your perception does not determine truth.

Worldly mindsets are based on perceptions that are not grounded in truth. They are based on feelings, assumptions, partial truths, and wrong judgments that are the result of influences that are opposed to God. Demons feed lies about God, ourselves, other people, and our circumstances into our minds. Every time they get us to swallow a lie and begin to act on and make choices based on the lie, another brick is added to the stronghold of an untruthful, worldly belief system.

No more lies

The problem is God doesn't do lies. His kingdom is founded in truth and only truth has a place in it. When we are first reconciled to God with heads filled with lies, distortions, and deception, he is not going to permit things to stay that way. He is not going to allow demonic, worldly influences to contaminate his relationship with us. If we are going to worship the God of truth we are going to have to part ways with lies:

> "Yet a time is coming and has now come when the true worshipers will worship the Father in spirit and truth, for they are the kind of worshipers the Father seeks. God is spirit and his worshipers must worship in spirit and in truth." (John 4: 23-24)

A lot of people worship God based on an image they have of him in their minds. Very often this image is not completely truthful. It's amazing how easy it is for us humans to adjust our notions of who God is and what he is like to suit ourselves. This is called idolatry – man creating a god according to his own imagination. There are many people in church who are worshiping a god who exists only in their minds.

In this passage God is saying our worship must be based on a truthful understanding of who he is and what he is like. We cannot worship him acceptably if our thinking about him and our attitudes towards him are not correct. We need to give up even dearly held beliefs if we find out they are not truthful and correct. God commands us to walk in truth. We are not allowed to believe whatever we want:

> "It has given me great joy to find some of your children walking in the truth, just as the Father commanded us." (2 John 4)

This is why change can be slow to come for some. It takes time to identify all the areas in our thinking that are not truthful. It takes time to come to grips with the degree of change we will need to make. Human beings are creatures of habit. We all like our comfort zones. Too many of us, however, have made ungodly mindsets and beliefs into a comfort zone. We like our beliefs because they are familiar and that gives us a sense of security.

My life was like this. My beliefs had me in a rut that was comfortable because it was familiar, not because I liked being there. I wanted change but I didn't want to have to change! Only when I was willing to admit I needed to change and began to make the effort did change begin to come.

We need God's manifest presence today more than ever

before and the world needs to see the reality of the kingdom of Heaven. It's so important that we begin to look at what might be hindering God's work and the place to start is with what is going on in our minds. God's blessing, favor, and power will only come to the degree that we are in agreement with him and his kingdom. Allow the Lord to renew your mind.

Take a closer look:

1. Take a moment right now to picture God in your mind. Is your idea of who and what he is accurate? How do you know?

2. Do you find yourself asking for prayer often so things in your life will change? Are they changing?

3. Are you stuck in repeating cycles of failure and defeat? If so, why do you think this is?

4. Are you secure in your beliefs about God, about yourself, about other people and about your circumstances? What evidence do you have that these beliefs are truthful and correct?

5. Have you ever experienced a change in your perception because you suddenly saw things from a different perspective? How did this affect your beliefs and behavior? Explain.

6. Do you think your "filter" needs to be cleaned?

2

Perception, Belief, and Choice

"My son, preserve sound judgment and discernment, do not let them out of your sight; they will
be life for you, an ornament to grace your neck.
Then you will go on your way in safety, and
your foot will not stumble." (Proverbs 3: 21-23)

As stated in the previous chapter, truth and perception are not the same thing. Truth exists apart from anyone's desire to believe it or not. Your belief does not create truth. Perception is what you see, or rather, what you think you see. However, what you think you see, or perceive, is not always the way things really are.

Perception can be influenced and distorted. It's like wearing a pair of glasses that are the wrong prescription, or seeing your reflection in a carnival mirror. If you didn't know the glasses were the wrong prescription or had never seen yourself in an ordinary mirror how would you know that the image you were seeing was distorted?

This is what my life was like before the Holy Spirit began to work in me. I just assumed that my life experiences, my thinking and beliefs were normal. I thought it was normal to be insecure and fearful. I thought it was normal to be depressed and negative, shy and withdrawn. It was all I had ever known.

I thought it was normal to have a hard time making friends, or to constantly worry about what others thought about me. I thought they saw me the same way I saw myself, as not good enough. I would interpret the words and behavior of others towards myself through my filter of negativity and self-rejection. It wasn't until later on when the Holy Spirit began to make me aware of the influences that had shaped my thinking that I began to see how much of my belief system was rooted in lies.

When I was in second grade the teacher gave me a job to do. I was to take all the partially filled containers of paint that we had used for an art project and combine the like colors together so we would have full containers instead of a bunch of partially filled ones. I misunderstood her. I thought she said to pour out all the paint in the partially filled containers.

When she saw that I had poured all her paint down the drain she got mad and yelled at me. I remember how bad and how stupid I felt. That day more lint got stuck in my filter. Because I didn't know truth, I didn't know how to process this experience in a godly way. It just reinforced the wrong thinking that was already filling my mind.

Your point of view

Perception is affected by your point of view. It's like the blind men who were trying to describe an elephant. One had a hold of the trunk and said elephants were long and flexible like snakes. Another was feeling the elephant's leg and said elephants were thick and round like tree trunks. Still another had a grip on the ear and said elephants were thin and flat like the sail on a boat. Each one's perception was distorted because their point of view was limited.

Because they were not able to see the whole picture, their conclusions were wrong. A partial truth that leads to wrong conclusions is just as bad as a lie. Our perception is a lot like this. We, as finite human beings are able to see only part of the picture when it comes to our lives and circumstances. We are limited by our physical senses and we often can only see what is right in front of our faces at any moment. So, a lot of the details that are required to make a truthful assessment of whatever might be happening to us escape us and we end up drawing wrong conclusions about things.

Have you ever had the experience of believing something that you later found out was not true? How did you feel when you found out the truth? Did you suddenly feel like someone had turned the lights on in your mind?

Every time you reach a wrong conclusion and it isn't corrected, it has the potential to become part of your belief system. As your belief system grows over time every new experience you have gets filtered through it.

If your belief system is full of wrong conclusions and assumptions your ability to see truth will be compromised. When a person has accepted a lie as the truth, he will see truth as a lie.

This is why we are told to be careful to preserve sound (truthful) judgment and discernment. We must make sure we are correctly processing all the input coming through our five senses, our emotions, our experiences etc. Only God is big enough to see the whole picture about anything we experience. In order for our judgment to be sound we will need to compare our perception with God's to make sure our discernment is correct.

God's point of view is the only one that is really truthful. This is why you need your Bible and the Spirit of God. They are where you go to so you can compare what you think you see to what is really true.

Potato or potahtoh?

We don't all see things the same. Take a look at this example: a man says to his wife, "I really don't deserve you." This statement can be taken two different ways. He could be saying his wife is such a wonderful blessing to him that he feels undeserving of having someone as terrific as she is. Or, he could be saying she is a horrible person and he can't see what he has done to deserve getting stuck with her. You can look at a glass of water that is filled halfway to the top and say it is half full or half empty. It is the "lint" in your filter that causes you to interpret what you see and hear one way or the other.

This is true even for something as trivial as choosing what to have for breakfast. You prefer Cheerios while another person likes oatmeal. You hate oatmeal because when your mom used to make it for you for breakfast she had a bad habit of burning it all the time. Every time you hear the word "oatmeal" it brings back the memory of the smell and taste of burned oatmeal. You do not consciously associate your hatred of oatmeal with your mother's poor cooking skills. To you oatmeal is just bad. So you refuse to eat it. And you never find out that oatmeal, properly cooked, can actually be good.

This is a silly example but it illustrates how our perceptions work. It shows how our perception is produced by how we process the things we experience. And it shows how perception can affect behavior and choice. Proverbs 23: 7 puts it this way:

"For as he thinketh in his heart, so is he." (KJV)

What people think about themselves, what they perceive about themselves, plays a larger role in determining the course of their lives than what is actually true about them. It is what you perceive, or what you think is true that will determine how you live and what choices you make.

A man who has been told from a very young age that he is stupid, or "bad" or a failure, will often incorporate this into his self-perception. He may be an absolute genius in fact. But he will be limited, often by his own choices, because his perception has been distorted. I see Christians like this all the time. They have a really hard time believing what God says about them because they have believed lies about themselves for such a long time. When you try to get some truth into their minds there is no room for it - there is too much lint in the filter and the air can't get through.

When I was in high school I really wanted to try out for the cheerleading squad. When I found out that the girls wanting to try out would have to perform their routines in front of the whole school, I couldn't muster the courage to do it. I was so fearful of failing and being rejected that there was no way I was going to risk putting myself in that spot.

As I look back, I can see today that there was really no reason to think that way. The only thing that kept me from what I wanted was my own mindset. It was a pattern that repeated itself over and over again during the course of my life. I didn't even bother to try to do many of the things I wanted to do because my fear of rejection and failure was too strong.

It is important that we come to the place where our belief systems are freed from lies and distortions so we once again process life through truth. When Saul was on the road to Damascus and saw Jesus, he was blinded (Acts 9). Ananias came and prayed for him. The Bible says when he laid his hands on Saul, "Immediately, something like scales fell from Saul's eyes, and he could see again" (verse 18).

I think what fell from his eyes was more than just the temporary blindness that came over him from seeing the brightness of the risen Lord. I think for the first time he could see and grasp the truth. Whatever had kept him from being able to recognize Jesus as the true Messiah, that had caused him to persecute Christians, fell off of his mind as well. He was now able to live his life in agreement with God's will because the blinders of his old beliefs and religious perceptions were now taken away. He was now able to see things from a new point of view, his perception was greatly altered, and, along with it, his behavior and choices.

This is the goal of correcting our perception and beliefs; so we can see in truth. Every day you act out your perceptions by making choices one way or another. Some of these choices are neutral, that is, they have no major impact on your life. Choosing Cheerios over oatmeal is a neutral choice.

I don't think God cares what you have for breakfast as long as it keeps you strong and healthy. But other choices have the power to determine where you end up in life. The decisions you make today set the stage for where you will be tomorrow. If these important choices are made based on how you perceive things isn't it important to know that what you are seeing is the way things really are?

Take the example of our man who was told he was stupid and a failure. Because he believes this he makes no effort to apply himself at school. He won't try because he thinks he is dumb and that there is no point in trying (and he is afraid if he tries, the words he has heard spoken about him will be proved true). He eventually drops out of school and accepts a low-paying, dead-end job because he is afraid he will fail if he tries to do more. He turns away from anything that looks like it might be hard. He misses out on God's purpose for his life, which was for him to become a successful, wealthy businessman who would use his wealth to finance God's kingdom work.

There are many Christians who find themselves in similar circumstances today. Because they let old, ungodly perceptions determine the choices they make they end up in continual cycles of aimless wandering and failure. Will power and good intentions alone will not deliver you. You must find the roots of the belief systems that are keeping you from seeing the truth about yourself, about God, about other people, and about your circumstances and purpose in life. Only when you are able to perceive the truth will you be able to make choices that are right and that bring you to the place God wants to put you.

In the next chapter we will talk about the influences that build our belief systems and where they come from.

Take a closer look:

1. Do you understand what perception is? How does perception influence belief?

2. Can you think of experiences you have had when what you thought was happening wasn't really what was happening? Give an example.

3. Have you ever made choices that turned out to be bad choices because your thinking at the time you made them wasn't correct?

4. Is what you believe about yourself true?

5. Have others said things to you or treated you in such a way that your self-perception has become distorted?

3

How Belief Systems Are Built

"Blessed are your eyes because they see, and
your ears because they hear." (Matthew 13: 16)

In the last chapter we talked about how perception
influences belief. What you think you see shapes your attitudes
and beliefs, which in turn cause you to make the choices you
make. Your choices produce consequences. If you make
choices that are foolish, sinful, and based on lies and deception,
you will reap misery, defeat, and failure. If you make choices
that are wise, based on God's kingdom truth you will reap
blessing, increase, peace and joy. Which would you rather
have?

In order to be able to sow properly you have to fix the thing
which motivates your choices - your thinking. Which means
you need to understand how you came to think the way you do
in the first place. Beliefs and perception are formed over time.
By the time you come a follower of Jesus you probably have
belief systems that are pretty well entrenched. This is why
those who get saved when they are younger seem to have an
easier time walking with God. There is less in the way of
habitual, wrong thinking that they have to deal with.

When you enter God's kingdom the stage is immediately

set for conflict. You find out rather quickly you have a lot of new stuff to learn. When you start to read the Bible it seems like much of what it says makes no sense. This is because the belief systems of the world and the belief system of the kingdom of God are not compatible.

You can't just add kingdom thinking and truth to the stuff that is already filling your mind. They don't get along and they won't mix. Old, untruthful, ungodly beliefs and perceptions must be uprooted to make way for new, truthful, godly beliefs and perceptions to take hold. Jesus said it this way:

> "No one sews a patch of unshrunk cloth on an old garment, for the patch will pull away from the garment making the tear worse. Neither do men pour new wine into old wineskins. If they do, the skins will burst, the wine will run out and the wineskins will be ruined. No, they pour new wine into new wineskins, and both are preserved." (Matthew 9: 16-17)

An old, worldly mindset cannot accommodate redeemed thinking. God cannot pour his new wine into an old wineskin that has been shaped and formed by old thinking. The wineskin (the thinking and mindset) must be new in order to be able to handle the new wine.

The system we call "the world" is made up of many institutions that all contribute to the formation of a mindset that is opposed to God and truth.

> "Once you were alienated from God and were enemies in your minds because of your evil behavior." (Colossians 1: 21)

We can use the terms "culture" and "identity" to describe what the influences of these institutions produce. It is through these cultural institutions that you learn what you are supposed to think and believe and how you should perceive and process the experiences you have in life.

These institutions are the sources of the influences that shaped your thinking before you became a follower of Jesus. They were not created by the devil. But, in a fallen world, the devil has warped what God created to accomplish his own purposes.

> "We know that we are children of God, and that the whole world is under the control of the evil one." (1 John 5: 19)

It is hard for us sometimes to think of these institutions as being in any way evil because they seem so familiar and normal to us. But when you begin to learn about God's kingdom ways, you realize a lot of what you thought was normal and right is not. Let's look at some of the major institutions of the world that shape beliefs and perceptions.

I. Family

Obviously, the devil did not create the family. But he has been busy using distorted family relationships and influences to ruin people's lives.

Unless you were born into a family where your parents were saved and filled with the knowledge of the truth, you most likely have experienced a family dynamic that was not what God intended. Often the influences that have been the most destructive in a person's life were those that came from other members of their family. Many people have no idea what a family ought to be or what a normal family (we are talking about what God says is normal) looks, or acts like.

Our families are the primary place where we learn how to deal with life. We gain our first sense of self in our families. We develop perspective on life; we learn how to deal with problems. We learn from our family, among other things, how relationships between different kinds of people work (father and mother, children and parents, brothers and sisters), the place God is to have in our lives (if any), how to treat other people, and what "right" and "wrong" are. We learn priorities and values that begin to determine the choices we make.

A lot of the ungodly thinking we must overcome first develops as we are growing up. Mom and Dad set examples for us, as do our brothers, sisters and grandparents, uncles, aunts etc. We receive from our generations (past and present) beliefs, attitudes, habits, and traditions. Everyone thinks that their own family is right or normal until they are given reason to question their family dynamic.

Family traditions, and thinking habits can be some of the hardest to change because people feel to change would be disloyal or that they would be saying their family is bad. The word "family" can extend to include your racial and cultural heritage as well as your flesh and blood relatives. Cultural traditions that are passed down through generations are not always godly and right. Many people have a "tribal" mentality where loyalty to their cultural or racial "tribe" takes first place above everything else. This presents a problem when we are confronted with the loyalty God requires of us as kingdom people.

Your family provides you with more than just biological DNA. You also receive spiritual DNA in the form of generational curses and spiritual influences that operate because of past sins and transgressions. These can have a huge influence on your life, especially if you are not aware they are there.

2. Education

The second source of influence that shapes thinking is education. I'm talking about things you learn in school, through the process of formal education, from preschool on up through graduate school and often beyond. You could include any place where some kind of instruction is taking place. It could be a religious school or whatever.

There is pressure to do well, and to be successful. This pressure is often what promotes the adoption of ideas and beliefs. The teachers are authority figures whom you are told you must please. Pleasing the teacher means giving them the "right" answer.

The influences that shape you in the educational system have the added advantage of the phenomena called "groupthink". When you get a large number of people together, most of them will want to fit in with the crowd. Being different from everyone else is uncomfortable. It doesn't really matter what the crowd thinks or does, what is important is being like everyone else and fitting in.

You can see the phenomena at work at any high school in the country. Kids will all dress the same, listen to the same music, use the same slang terms in their communication, cut their hair the same etc. This is also called peer-pressure. People want to be accepted by their peers and whatever the philosophy of the moment is that is popular with their peer group they will most likely adopt.

It is among a crowd of our peers that most of us develop a sense of our place in life, where we fit in, or whether we fit in at all. Often it is not just what you learn in the classroom but what you perceive as you relate within your peer group in the educational system that forms your beliefs and thinking patterns.

The educational system is also where you are exposed to new ideas and perceptions. College campuses especially are known for being breeding grounds of social change, unrest, and rebellion – think U.C. Berkeley. People find their beliefs challenged as they are presented with new information and ideas. Some people just add new ideas to the pile that already fills their heads without realizing many of these new ideas are not compatible with things they say they already believe.

3. Media

What I mean by "media" are the channels through which a lot of the information we receive comes. Things like television, radio, books, newspapers, magazines, the internet, social media, etc. Many would like to believe that what they receive through the media is unbiased and completely truthful. To think this is to be naïve. What comes through the media will be a reflection of the people who control the media.

Anyone who knows anything about history knows that channels of communication have often been used and controlled by people who have an agenda to push. This is called propaganda. Information is selectively presented to manipulate people's perception and beliefs to make them conform with those of whoever controls the media. The agenda being pushed could be something as simple as trying to get you to leave your car at home and take public transit to work. Or, it could be presenting information about the candidates in an election in such a way as to swing people's support from one candidate to the other.

It doesn't matter what your personal political or social beliefs are; when information is withheld or selectively presented to manipulate people's perception it is deceitful. The use of deception to promote certain kinds of thinking does not come from God.

Think about the information that comes to you through the media. Would it ever occur to you to question or doubt someone who seems as nice and sincere as the local news anchor on the 6:00 p.m. news broadcast? And you don't have to be talking about willful deception. The anchorperson may think all the news s/he is presenting is right and correct. That doesn't make it truthful. There are many voices coming at us through the media telling us they are the ones who are right or who have the truth. Remember Pilate's response to Jesus in John 18: 37-38:

> "Jesus answered, "You are right in saying I am a king. In fact, for this reason I was born, and for this I came into the world, to testify to the truth. Everyone on the side of truth listens to me." "What is truth?" Pilate asked.

Pilate was confused about what the truth was. There were so many voices in his day, all proclaiming to be the truth he didn't know which one to listen to. This doesn't mean you should be paranoid and constantly suspicious. It just means you must remember who controls the media and not blindly believe whatever you are told.

4. Entertainment

People go to a movie or watch a show on T.V. or go to a concert to relax and enjoy the presentation. A lot of entertainment is just that – entertainment. Some of it, though, is just another way peoples' perceptions and beliefs are manipulated and directed.

The way characters are portrayed in a movie or on television has a lot of influence on the way people perceive those kinds of people in the real world. There has been a lot of change in the field of entertainment in the last 50 years or so. Movies and television are not really that old. People have been concerned that what we see should more accurately reflect what they call "real life". Some of this is good. Instead of there being only white, Caucasian characters, we now have characters of practically every race and nationality. But some of what passes for entertainment is really just propaganda in disguise.

People have discovered that when you go to the movies, or watch T.V. you let your guard down a little. You are just there to passively receive whatever is presented. So, often characters and plots are designed to present whatever social, religious, or political perspective the scriptwriters and producer want. The influence is often subtle (but not always). And, over time, repeated again and again, peoples' ideas and values can be shaped and changed.

Entertainment has become very important in our culture. We are obsessed with celebrities and urged to copy them, to want what they want and to live like they live. This includes sports celebrities. After all, sports are just another form of entertainment. The amount of time and money that is spent on entertainment is a reflection of how important it is to people.

People seem to live vicariously through their favorite celebrities. Their own lives look dull and boring in comparison. The more people are caught up in entertainment, the harder it is to deal with the truth of real life. Too much fantasy and escapism can warp our thinking where we may begin to lose the ability to differentiate between reality and unreality.

Children especially are vulnerable because they tend not to question what they are presented with. Think about the phenomena of video games. Kids are introduced to witchcraft, sexual sin and perversion, and violence, all of which are made to seem harmless and innocent because they come packaged as "fun".

5. Government

Government shapes our thinking and perception in many ways. Law and policy, what we are and are not allowed to do or say, will depend on the worldview of whoever happens to be writing it. In some countries, personal freedoms are practically nonexistent because of the worldview of those who govern. This includes restriction on what is acceptable belief and speech.

Some countries severely restrict the information their citizens are allowed to have access to, including information about what is happening in other parts of the world. People living in countries like these often have a distorted view of the world (think North Korea). Every government uses its power and influence to direct the lives of its citizens in the direction it thinks is right and proper. We call this social engineering. Certain behaviors are rewarded; others are not.

Think of how the habit of smoking has fallen into disrepute over the years. Someone decided that smoking was a bad habit and used governmental power and influence, through restrictive laws about where and when you could smoke (and how much it will cost) to push people to give it up altogether. Things such as the tax code, zoning restrictions, environmental laws, laws restricting business, commerce, and immigration are utilized by whoever is in power to lead (or drive) people towards certain kinds of thinking and behavior.

Making something illegal goes a long way towards changing the way people think and behave. There are places where it is illegal to be a Christian or to convert to Christianity, or to say anything against the things Christianity says are wrong. In the name of multiculturalism, political correctness, and "fairness", governments make it illegal to speak truth to culture.

6. Business and commerce

Business and commerce have to do with creating, buying, and selling goods and services. It's about the creation of wealth. We engage in business and commerce whenever we sell something or buy something. Business is what provides most people with their living. They earn money to support themselves and their families. It is what takes up the largest portion of our time during the day.

Because it's where their money comes from, people tend to give a lot of time and attention to their jobs. A lot of their thinking centers on how to do well at work, how they can get a better job, how to earn more money, or how to get everything done that their job requires them to get done. There can be great pressure to go along to get along, even with things they may not think are right.

Businesses will resort to questionable tactics because they think they won't be able to compete if they don't. The world's system of business will try to tell you that you won't succeed if you do things God's way. Jobs can often be so demanding that other important areas of life get neglected. People will give work priority because they are afraid if they don't, they will lose their job and have no money to pay their bills.

The acquisition of wealth is what most people think and

worry about. People will do crazy things if they think they might be in danger of losing their money or if they think they are not getting enough of it.

Marketing is a large part of business. Marketing is all about getting people to want to buy your stuff. Marketing appeals to greed and envy. It is directed at the lust of the flesh, lust of the eyes and pride of life. People will spend money they don't have to buy something they don't need because someone told them they are supposed to want it.

The world's system of business will try to lure you into lifestyles and behaviors that are not in agreement with kingdom values. If you buy into the thinking of the world, that you can't be happy or fulfilled or accepted unless you have certain stuff or "enough" money, you're going to have a hard time living for God.

7. Religion

It's easy to see how religion affects our belief systems. Religion is about how you relate to God. People tend to listen when they believe someone is speaking to them on God's behalf.

It's hard to change religious thinking. In the back of our minds we worry that we might be offending God if we stop believing in our religious traditions. By its very nature, religious indoctrination tends to keep people trapped because of what is at stake – eternity. Religion is also what people know the least about. For most people it tends to be shrouded in mystery.

Religion is presided over by men and women who are supposed to know about God (or the supreme deity or deities), and how to make him (it, them) happy. So we tend to let them tell us what to believe and rarely question what we are told.

Religious systems often make it impossible for the average person to find out for him or herself what is really true about their religion. The religion's holy scriptures are often written and spoken in holy languages that are known only to the initiated. Only certain persons are qualified to learn the holy scriptures and languages and explain them so the rest of us must just rely on what we are told.

Religions are about performance; doing rather than being. They are comprised of rules and regulations that are supposed to earn the religious practitioner favor as they (the rules) are religiously obeyed. Even simple faith can be turned into a religious work when it becomes just another way of performing in order to get something from God or to earn his love and approval. You can tell religion by its fruit: pride, false humility, self-righteousness, an unteachable spirit, and a hard heart.

All kinds of strange thinking and behavior are the result of religion. It almost seems the stranger it is the more likely people are to believe it.

That was then

All these institutions have had a hand in shaping our perception, belief, and identity. Because they are to a greater or lesser degree (depending on what time in history it is) under the influence of the kingdom of darkness they produce people who are loyal to the world, its values and priorities, which are the values and priorities of the kingdom of darkness. Until we come to Christ our perceptions and beliefs are formed by the world. When we believe in the Lord, the Holy Spirit begins the process of renewing our minds. Old, worldly, untruthful thinking is like a veil over the mind. It must be removed so we can accept and live in truth.

Take a closer look:

1. Think about the institutions we have just talked about. How have your perceptions and beliefs been affected by them?

2. What are some ways your thinking has been shaped by your family?

3. How did your experience in the educational system affect your beliefs and define your identity?

4. Have you ever felt pressure through the media to think or see things a certain way?

5. What religious traditions did you grow up with? How have they affected the way you related to God today?

6. How has the world of entertainment affected your perceptions and beliefs?

7. List any other ways you can think of how your beliefs and perceptions have been formed by these institutions.

4

Tearing Down, Building Up

> "He replied, "If you have faith as small as a mustard seed, you can say to this mulberry tree, 'Be uprooted and planted in the sea,' and it will obey you." (Luke 17: 6)

As we saw in the last chapter, our belief systems are formed by the world before we are born again. As such, they reflect the world, and the world's thinking and priorities. God's kingdom is opposed to the world. The Apostle John tells us that whoever loves the world is opposed to God:

> "Do not love the world or anything in the world. If anyone loves the world, the love of the Father is not in him. For everything in the world – the cravings of sinful man, the lust of his eyes and the boasting of what he has and does – comes not from the Father but from the world." (1 John 2: 15-16)

We are not to be like the world. Our worldview, perspective, priorities, and beliefs should reflect the fact we are new creations in Christ Jesus where old things, including old mindsets and beliefs, are passed away.

"Therefore come out from them and be separate, says the Lord. Touch no unclean thing, and I will receive you. I will be a Father to you, and you will be my sons and daughters, says the Lord Almighty." (2 Corinthians 6: 17-18)

The institutions of the world produce people with mindsets and belief systems that are not in agreement with God. And, as we noted earlier, renewing your mind is not just a matter of adding new ideas and information to what you have already accumulated. A new belief system, like any structure must have a proper foundation on which to be built.

When someone wants to build a new structure the first thing they do is clear the ground of any old, decrepit structures that may be occupying the space they want to build on. Then, a new foundation must be laid that will be strong enough to support whatever is to be built.

"Then the LORD reached out his hand and touched my mouth and said to me, "Now I have put my words in your mouth. See, today I appoint you over nations and kingdoms to uproot and tear down, to destroy and to overthrow, to build and to plant." (Jeremiah 1: 9-10)

Notice the process here. Which comes first? The tearing down and uprooting must come before the building and the planting. Ungodly, untruthful beliefs must be uprooted so truth can come in and take their place.

The Bible tells us that Jesus Christ, the knowledge of him as Savior and Lord, his resurrection from the dead, and what he did for us on the cross, is the foundation upon which all else is built for the believer. Truth begins and ends in Jesus Christ.

He is the way, the truth and the life. Any mindset or belief system that does not or cannot agree with this must be uprooted and discarded.

A belief system can be equated with what we call a stronghold. A stronghold is a fortified place, usually surrounded by walls, with guards protecting it. Strongholds in your mind are made up of beliefs and perceptions. They can be one of two kinds.

If your beliefs are truthful and correct, the stronghold in your mind will be like a fortress, a place where you are protected from your enemies and their attacks (remember the devil uses lies as his ammunition).

If your beliefs are erroneous, distorted, and untrue the stronghold in your mind will be like a prison. The wrong beliefs will act like a prison cell keeping you locked up away from the freedom and blessing God has for you. Demons (guarding the stronghold) will exploit your wrong beliefs to keep you from recognizing and experiencing God's love, favor, and goodness.

The difference between being in a place of protection or being in jail is the nature of the beliefs that create your belief system. Many Christians are surprised to learn that the enemy has set up structures in their minds that enable him to maintain an entrenched position in their lives.

Tear down the old

By the time you are born again, the devil has had a lot of time to build his structures in your thinking. Every lie, deception, half-truth, or wrong judgment that you accept becomes part of that structure. And, once you accept a lie, your ability to recognize truth is diminished. You become susceptible to more lies and deception. They build on each other.

Take the example of a person who has been hurt by rejection. When a person believes no one loves or wants them, every word and action from other people will be interpreted in light of this belief.

Relationships and trust will be difficult for this person because they are operating from a core belief that no one really loves or wants them. If you try to say something nice to them or show them some kind of love or attention they will most likely respond with suspicion: "What do you really want?"

The person may begin to believe that nothing about them is good enough. After all, if they were good enough people would love them. The person might begin to distance themself from others. They will do this believing they are only protecting themselves from bad people.

Or they might become passive people pleasers, trying to get others to love them by giving them what they want. They may believe God has rejected them too and begin to resent him for it, or go to extremes to try to earn God's approval.

As this ungodly belief system is built in their minds they find themselves more and more shut off from God and other people. Their beliefs have effectively created a jail from which they cannot escape.

The only way to get out of the jail is to change the beliefs that create the jail. How do I know this? I know it because this is the way I used to think. Rejection thinking controlled my life. Everything that happened to me, all the words I heard were filtered through this thinking. Spirits of rejection worked overtime in my mind to make sure I stayed in my jail.

These are the kinds of belief structures that must be torn down before God's truth and love can truly be established in a person's life. The Bible says darkness and light cannot co-exist (2 Corinthians 6:14). The kingdom of truth and light cannot be built alongside or co-mingled with a kingdom of darkness and deception.

You cannot serve two masters. It is not truthful to say no one loves you or cares about you. Until you have met every single person on the face of the earth and they have all rejected you it is wrong to say no one loves you. And even then, God loves you. So the belief no one loves you, or cares about you is a lie.

Changing your beliefs will free you from the jail as long as the new beliefs you acquire are truthful and correct. We are told that getting rid of ungodly thinking is the way to demolish the structures the devil has built in our lives:

> "For though we live in the world, we do not wage war as the world does. The weapons we fight with are not the weapons of the world. On the contrary, they have divine power to demolish strongholds. We demolish arguments and every pretension that sets itself up against the knowledge of God, and we take captive every thought to make it obedient to Christ." (2 Corinthians 10: 3-5)

Build the new

Every thought, belief, and argument that is contrary to the truth of Christ and the word of God must be torn down and our thoughts and beliefs must be taken captive, that is, brought into agreement with truth. This brings us to the second part of tearing down and building up.

After the tearing down something must be built to take the place of what was torn down. It is not enough to discard old thinking. You need to replace old beliefs with new ones. A new structure must be built to take the place of the old one. The tearing down and overthrowing must be followed with building and planting.

As new, truthful beliefs are acquired and established, new walls are built. These walls, however, are built out of truth. Truth is the defense you have against the weapons of the enemy, which are lies and deception (Ephesians 6). Familiarity with the truth will enable you to recognize lies before you are ensnared by them.

When your mind is filled with truth and your beliefs are grounded in truth you will no longer be a sitting duck for the enemy to come and pick off. Your new belief system will create a place of protection and refuge where you will be able to find peace and rest.

Sometimes it is painful to learn the truth about things. Lies can create a comfort zone of counterfeit peace that the devil won't disturb. He will let you have your "peace" if it means he can keep you in your jail.

A lot of people prefer to remain in their comfort zone of counterfeit peace. They don't want to deal with the truth. It's hard for these people to walk with God because he won't co-exist with lies. And there is no middle ground where God will agree to let you hang on to some lies and believe some truth.

The old structures of the past must be demolished to make way for the work of the Holy Spirit as he builds his own structures in your life. This work of tearing down and building up goes on simultaneously. The work can only proceed, however, if you allow it.

A choice must be made to come out of agreement with wrong thinking that the Holy Spirit points out to you. He cannot dismantle old beliefs without your permission and agreement. And, he cannot build new belief structures without your participation and agreement. You must make the choice to allow him to renew your mind if you want to live out God's purpose for your life.

Take a closer look:

1. Ask the Holy Spirit to show you any "old" beliefs that still guide your life today. What are they?

2. Do you recognize the Holy Spirit working in your life to renew your mind? Give an example.

3. What areas of your belief system is the Holy Spirit talking to you about?

4. Do you understand that renewing your mind requires your active participation? Explain.

5. Or are you sitting around waiting for God to somehow "change" things?

5

Wrong Beliefs about God

> "Jesus Christ is the same yesterday and today
> and forever." (Hebrews 13:8)

This is the first of four areas of belief we are going to look at so you can begin to identify where your beliefs are not truthful. The first is truth about God.

It is important to know you are believing what is true about God. If you are serving a god who is merely a creation of your imagination, or a creation built of lies, deception, or half-truths, it is idolatry.

> "You shall not make for yourself an image in
> the form of anything in heaven above or on the
> earth beneath or in the waters below." (Exodus
> 20: 4)

Images are not just statues. Images can reside in the mind too. You carry an image of what you think God is like in your mind. And we often imagine God as we want him to be, not as he really is.

Much of our struggle in our relationship with God is understanding who he is and what he is really like; his

45

character, person, and his motives towards us. We have trouble because we often believe things about God that are not true and question his character of love and goodness. We are not sure we can trust him to keep his promises. We are not so sure his will is good and good for us. We are afraid if we obey him we will miss out on all the good things in life.

Satan is more than happy to supply you with all kinds of ideas about God that make him look bad and that keep you at a distance from him. Often demon spirits attempt to impersonate the Holy Spirit. People listen to them thinking they are listening to God. These demons try to pervert your understanding of God because they don't want you finding out what God is really like.

The first untruthful beliefs you need to confront and deal with are the ones you have about God. If you don't have a correct perception of him, and truthful beliefs about who he is and the place he is to have in your life, nothing else will be right. Jesus said:

> "So do not worry, saying, 'What shall we eat?' or 'What shall we drink?' or 'What shall we wear?' For the pagans run after all these things, and your heavenly Father knows that you need them. But seek first his kingdom and his righteousness, and all these things will be given to you as well." (Matthew 6: 31-33)

Seeking first the kingdom means to make it your top priority in life to gain knowledge and understanding of God and to live in right relationship with him. Everything else in your life will be determined by whether or not you are doing this. You can't be in right relationship with God if you don't know the truth about him.

The truth about God

The place you go to find the truth about God is the Bible. When you read it you need to let it speak for itself instead of reading into it what you want to hear. The Bible tells you who God is, his true character, and the purpose of his relationship with you.

You learn that God is holy, just, pure and sinless, good, kind, merciful and loving, and that he cannot and will not tolerate sin and evil forever. You learn he is absolute ruler of the universe, creator and sustainer of all, and that he requires you to swear allegiance to him as King and Lord in the person of Christ Jesus. You read about how he made a way for you to be restored to himself through the sacrifice of Jesus on the cross.

You learn about the terms of the covenant that govern your relationship with him. You learn that he loves you absolutely and unconditionally and that you can't earn his love or blessings; they are freely given to those who choose to walk in covenant relationship with him. You learn God is not a big old man sitting up on a cloud in heaven wringing his hands over the misdeeds of the people of the earth. He is not motivated by a bad temper or hurt feelings. He is constant, consistent, and unchangeable.

Many of our wrong beliefs about God come from what we hear from other people. Family and cultural religious traditions and generational religious influences can color your perception of God and cause you to believe things about him that are not true.

If you were raised in a strict religious home or with certain religious traditions you might have a hard time believing God to be kind and gentle, or that he is personally interested in you. You might think you have to earn things from him by being good. Remember how Jesus said it was the religious traditions of the Pharisees that shut the door of the kingdom to those who wanted to come in (Matthew 23: 13). Religious beliefs that rely heavily on sets of rules or performance (doing good deeds etc), to earn God's love and approval can be hard to uproot. People are often afraid to let go of them.

Sometimes we allow people to influence our perception of God by their own personal experiences. We will judge God on the basis of what others say about their experiences of his love, faithfulness, and goodness. How many times have you heard people say God is not good because he allows bad things to happen in the world? And many of them have never personally had any of these bad experiences happen to them. They are only repeating what they have heard someone else say.

Popular culture, the media, television and movies, and other influences also have the power to shape our beliefs about God if we let them. There have been many movies and T.V. shows where Christians were depicted as weird, dishonest and deceitful, out of touch with reality, or untrustworthy, or where the idea of believing in God is mocked and ridiculed or even made to look dangerous. God is made to look bad by making his followers look bad. (And often his followers look bad because they believe stuff about God that isn't true.)

Another way people develop wrong ideas about God is when they project on him the experiences they have had with other people. For example, a person who had an angry, abusive father might have a hard time relating to a God called Father because all they know about fathers is what they have experienced with their own human father.

Or, if a person has suffered in some way at the hand of the authority figures in their life they might have difficulty relating to God because they see him as another authority figure and assume he is like the rest of them. Perhaps they have experienced broken promises and disappointment from these authority figures, or even abuse, and they unconsciously expect to experience the same from God. This is especially true when these authority figures are religious authority figures.

We can't let our ideas and beliefs about God be determined by anything other than truth. We cannot allow the subjective experiences of other people alone to determine what we believe.

Is God good?

Another problem we have believing the truth about God is we have different meanings for the words used to describe him.

> "As Jesus started on his way, a man ran up to him and fell on his knees before him. "Good teacher," he asked, "what must I do to inherit eternal life?" "Why do you call me good?" Jesus answered. "No one is good – except God alone." (Mark 10: 17-18)

The rich young man called Jesus good. In his mind certain beliefs and expectations were attached to this word. He discovered however that God's definition of "good" was not the same as his. When he found out that God's good for him was to sell everything he had and give it to the poor, he seems to have changed his mind about Jesus being good.

The same thing happens to us. We have ideas about what it means to love or what it means to be kind and good, or just or fair. When God's definitions of these things do not match our own we are disappointed and have a hard time believing God

49

is good, kind, just, or fair.

Our idea of good usually means what's good for me, or what I want. Our definition of what love is and how it should be demonstrated may not be the same as God's. We think if he loves us he will give us whatever we want, never let us experience anything unpleasant or painful, and never expect more of us than we feel like giving. When you see God use certain words to describe what he is like you need to make sure that your definitions of those words are the same as the ones he uses.

Here are some examples of wrong beliefs about God:

1. God doesn't (or can't) love me

2. God is what I imagine him to be.

3. Everyone's ideas about who or what God is are valid.

4. If I trust God he will let me down (like people do).

5. God doesn't get involved in the day-to-day details of our lives. He has more important things to do.

6. God needs me to be good (he will be diminished in some way if I am not).

7. If I pray more and go to church more and read my Bible more God will love me more.

8. God doesn't care how I feel.

9. God can't be good because (fill in the blank with some evil thing that has or is happening in the world).

10. God is just like people only bigger.

11. There is no God.

12. God must be approached through certified religious figures. I can't just go talk to him myself.

Take a closer look:

1. Are your beliefs about God correct and truthful?   How do you know?

2. Where were your beliefs about God acquired?

3. Have any of your beliefs about God changed over time? In what way?

4. Do you ever find yourself unconsciously attributing to God the same faults and flaws you have seen in people?

5. Do you believe God is good?

6. Does your opinion of God's goodness change when your circumstances change?

7. Do you find yourself concentrating on those aspects of God's person and character that you like and ignoring those you don't?

8. Do you fear God? What does it mean to you to fear God? Is it right to fear God?

9. What does the Bible say about who God is and what he is like? Write down below some scriptures that talk about what God is like:

6

Beliefs About Ourselves

"Do you not realize that Christ Jesus is in you?"
(2 Corinthians 13:5)

Almost as effective as getting us to believe lies about God is getting us to believe lies about ourselves. Remember how we said earlier that what is true about you has less of an effect on your life than what you believe to be true. When you believe lies about yourself it's hard to mature as a follower of Jesus.

Your time in the world has caused you to acquire wrong beliefs about your true character and personality, strengths, and weaknesses. You probably have a habit of seeing yourself through the filter of past experiences rather than through the truth of God's word. God cannot work with you when you can't or won't see the truth about yourself. Maturity means having the ability to truthfully assess your character and behavior.

Having truthful beliefs mean you have an accurate assessment of your person and character, both your strengths and weaknesses. If you have ever watched the show "American Idol" on TV you have probably seen examples of people who had trouble truthfully assessing themselves. There have been many people on the show who were convinced they were very talented when they really had no talent at all, and refused to listen to the truth about themselves when told.

Truthful beliefs means you don't think more highly or more lowly of yourself than you ought. You should neither exaggerate nor diminish what you really are.

> "For by the grace given me I say to every one of you: Do not think of yourself more highly than you ought, but rather with sober judgment, in accordance with the measure of faith God has given you." (Romans 12: 3)

Here Paul is telling the Romans to have sober judgment when it comes to thinking about themselves. What happens to your judgment when you are not sober? Have you ever seen a person who was intoxicated or high on drugs? What happens to their judgment?

People who are drunk cannot judge anything correctly. They think they are being funny and clever when they are really being irritating and annoying. They can be rude, abusive, exhibit questionable behavior, and be totally unaware of the true nature of they are doing. Often when they sober up and are told how they behaved while they were drunk, they have a hard time believing it or they don't remember anything at all. When people use drugs it interferes with their ability to tell the real world from fantasy. Drug users often believe they can jump off a ten-story building and fly, or eat poison and it won't kill them.

The influences of drugs and alcohol keep people from exercising sober, that is, truthful judgment. Your experiences in the world before you are saved can have the same effect as drugs and alcohol. Your judgment will be impaired if you are still under the influence of past life experiences and the belief system you acquired from life lived in a world without the true knowledge of God. When you are born again, the Holy Spirit begins the process of sobering you up.

Here are some examples of wrong beliefs about yourself:

1. I'll never succeed.

2. I don't need God in order to be a good person.

3. I can't forgive

4. If I fail, it means I'm worthless.

5. I am not lovable.

6. I'm fine just the way I am (said in response to someone pointing out a character flaw)

8. I can't tell people the truth about myself.

9. My flaws and imperfections must be covered up and hidden.

10. I need to fit in and be accepted, whatever the cost.

11. It's my job to fix others or make them happy.

12. If I don't take care of #1 no one else will.

13. My feelings are a reliable guide for my life.

Correcting beliefs about yourself can be more difficult than correcting beliefs about God because a lot of us have blind spots; we can't see where our beliefs are wrong. To have to re-adjust your thinking about yourself can be hard. It can be humbling to find out the truth about yourself. It can be humbling but it is also liberating.

Correcting your self-perception may require you to listen to people who know you, who can see those things about you that you either can't or don't want to see. And this doesn't just mean flaws and weaknesses. Some people have a harder time believing good things about themselves than bad.

When you confront your beliefs about yourself you may need to learn to see people and past life experiences from a new perspective. You might need to admit you were wrong in the way you responded to the words and behaviors of other people.

In order to correct our beliefs we need to be able to look at some kind of picture, or pattern that shows what we are supposed to think. Again, we go to the Bible to find it:

> "For the word of God is living and active. Sharper than any double-edged sword, it penetrates even to dividing soul and spirit, joints and marrow; it judges the thoughts and attitudes of the heart." (Hebrews 4: 12)

The word of God, illuminated by the Holy Spirit, the one who leads you and guides you into all truth, will show you what you are really like. If you are listening, you can hear the Holy Spirit talk to you about your beliefs, behaviors, and attitudes as you read and hear the word.

> "Do not merely listen to the word and so deceive yourselves. Do what is says. Anyone who listens to the word but does not do what it says is like a man who looks at his face in a mirror and, after looking at himself, goes away

and immediately forgets what he looks like."
(James 1: 22-24)

The word of God is a mirror that reveals what you are really like when you put it into practice. When you try to do what it says your true character and person will be revealed. For example, when you see the command "love your neighbor as yourself", what kind of response does it produce from you? That response will tell you what you are really like.

At the same time, this mirror of the word shows what you are becoming. It is the pattern of what God's covenant people are to be and shows you how to think, how to act, and how to relate to the world and the people in it.

Take a closer look:

1. Are your beliefs about yourself truthful and correct? How do you know?

2. Have you ever had someone try to talk to you about things they see in you that you don't see? These could be good qualities, not just flaws. How did you respond?

3. What are some of the beliefs about yourself that the Holy Spirit has changed over time?

4. Are you able to admit your faults and weaknesses or do you get defensive when someone points them out?

5. Are you able to admit to your strengths and abilities without getting puffed up or do you find yourself minimizing them?

6. In what ways should you think more highly of yourself than you do now? In what ways should you think more humbly of yourself than you do now?

7. What does God's word say about you? Write some examples below:

_____

_____

_____

_____

_____

_____

_____

_____

_____

_____

_____

_____

7

Beliefs About Other People

"'Love your neighbor as yourself." (Mark 12:31)

People are the focus of God's kingdom business here on earth. People are what's important to God. In order to bring a harvest into the kingdom you have to interact with people. Relationship is how the kingdom grows and expands. Relationships are how love is given and received.

The devil works hard to hinder and ruin relationships to keep the kingdom of heaven from being expressed here on earth. He does this by getting us to judge people falsely, and make assumptions about them that are not true, or to take what we know to be true and respond to it the wrong way.

We often make judgments about people's motives, intentions, and character without really knowing them. We make assumptions about their behavior, why they do the things they do. And most people are harsher in their assessments of others than they ever are of themselves.

Such judgments often result in stereotypes, bigotry, prejudice, and conditional love, or in thinking more highly or lowly of people than they really deserve. All of which keep us from having truthful relationships. You can't relate to people effectively if you don't know or won't believe the truth about them.

Often our first perceptions of people come from what we see on the outside. We look at how they are dressed, whether or not they take care of themselves, are clean, well-groomed etc. (according to the standards we consider right or proper) and make a judgment about what kind of person they are. Or we look at what race they are, or hear what language they are speaking, whether or not they have an accent. We listen and decide whether or not they fit in or belong.

We see how old they are, or whether or not they seem to be friendly, and decide if we want to relate to them in any way. If people manage to get past the first round of judgments, we will then make judgments based on whether or not they meet our expectations, or based on their behavior towards us or towards other people. The problem is we often process our experiences with other people through our own set of filters that causes us to wrongly interpret their words, or actions.

Suppose you shop at a certain grocery store. You notice one of the workers at the check out stand seems to have a frown on her face all the time. As you shop there over a period of weeks and months this person hardly ever smiles and is often short of temper and unfriendly. You eventually decide she is rude and cranky and may even think about no longer shopping at a store that would employ someone like her.

What you don't know is she caught her husband cheating on her and that he is in the process of divorcing her. Her kids are acting out because of all the stress in the home and her health is suffering because of the whole experience. She feels betrayed and the load of anger she is carrying around is spilling over into her interactions with other people.

You yourself feel very uncomfortable around people like her because your own past experiences have made you very sensitive to any kind of negativity. Because you struggle with past experiences of rejection, you interpret her behavior as rejection towards yourself and you take her rudeness and unfriendliness personally even though it has nothing to do with you.

We must be very careful when we are around people not to judge or make assumptions about them too quickly. It takes time to get to know someone well enough to know what is really inside them. We have to make sure we are not projecting our own negative experiences on others and that we are not interpreting their words and actions the wrong way.

> "Stop judging by mere appearances, and make a right judgment." (John 7: 24)

We need to make sure we don't allow only appearances and what we see on the surface to determine what we think about people. We must allow for what we cannot see, inside the person's heart and mind where we cannot go, and let the Holy Spirit confirm the beliefs we form about others.

> "Do not judge, or you too will be judged. For in the same way you judge others, you will be judged, and with the measure you use, it will be measured to you." (Matthew 7:1)

What is he saying here? I believe Jesus is telling us that we are not to hold others to standards that we don't hold ourselves to. Much of what we believe about people has to do with how we see them act and behave. Because people are usually much harder on the faults of others than they are on their own faults, they expect more from other people than they expect from themselves. We tend to want to excuse our own bad behavior and want others to excuse it too, but we are less willing to excuse their bad behavior.

Jesus is saying we will be held to the same standard we hold others to, so we must be careful to make sure the beliefs we form about others are based on truth, just as we want others to believe the truth about us. Here are some examples of wrong beliefs about others.

1. People (or men or women in particular) can't be trusted. (blanket judgments)

2. If others would change then I could or would too. (Other people are responsible for your success or happiness.)

3. Human beings are inherently good.

4. They need to meet my expectations before I love them.

5. People aren't worth the trouble it takes to get to know them.

6. If I let them get close to me they will take advantage of me. (another blanket judgment.)

7. They will never change. (Not allowing that people can change over time.)

8. I know what they are thinking. (Making assumptions according to your own pre-conceived notions.)

It's not wrong to form beliefs and opinions about other people. We are told in 1 Corinthians that we are to supposed to judge others in the church, that is, we are supposed to judge their actions as conforming to righteousness or not. Chapter 5 tells about the man who was having sexual relations with his father's wife (his stepmother). Paul told the church they should expel this man. The Corinthian church had been unwilling to make a judgment about him:

> "What business is it of mine to judge those outside the church? Are you not to judge those inside? God will judge those outside. "Expel the wicked man from among you." (v. 12-13)

Having truthful beliefs about people means we correctly (as far as we are able) assess their entire character, not just the parts we like or admire. There have been a lot of people who have been taken in by charisma and personality, or who were so impressed by talent and skill that no thought was given to truthfully assessing character.

Perhaps you like sports. Because you like sports and are impressed by those who possess skill and great ability when it comes to sports, you are inclined to overlook anything about your sports heroes that might be unpleasant. If a man is good at batting a ball or throwing a pass, he must be a good guy, right?

Or, maybe you like movies. If a person is a good actor and you like all the characters she portrays in the movies, she herself must be just like the characters she portrays, right? Or you are a faithful church-goer. A preacher comes to your church and preaches a rousing sermon that has everyone on their feet cheering and shouting. The preacher must be a godly person if everyone responded so enthusiastically to the sermon, right? Having truthful beliefs about people means looking past what appeals to you (or not) and withholding judgment until you have enough information to judge correctly.

Obviously, there is a limit to what you can find out about people. There are those you interact with who you don't see often enough to be able to get to know them really well. There are those who display false personality traits, which makes it difficult to find out the truth about them.

The point is we need to leave room for adjustment in our beliefs about people. We must allow that people can change and keep in mind that until we know everything about them, we may have to adjust our beliefs about them from time to time as we acquire more information. We must make sure we want to know the truth about them and not be content with superficial judgments and assumptions. We must make the effort, as much as we are able, to find out what is true and not let our own weaknesses color our judgments of others.

There is one thing about others that we are not to judge - people's hearts. We can judge their actions. But until they reveal their own hearts it is impossible for us to know apart from the Holy Spirit revealing things to us. We are not to lock people up with our judgments.

Take a closer look:

1. Are your beliefs about other people correct and truthful?

2. Do you have any prejudices? What are they? How did you acquire them?

3. How have you allowed your own personal experiences to influence the way you relate to and judge others?

4. Are you satisfied with superficial assumptions about people or do you make reasonable efforts to know the truth about them?

5. Should what we believe about people change the way we

treat them?

6. Below, write down some scriptures that talk about how we should think and behave towards others:

_____

_____

_____

_____

_____

_____

_____

_____

_____

_____

_____

_____

_____

_____

8

Beliefs About Our Life and Circumstances

"And we know in all things God works for the good of those who love him . . ." (Romans 8: 28)

If you don't have correct, truthful beliefs about the things that happen to you (good and bad) and why your life is the way it is, it is going to be hard to respond and deal with those circumstances correctly. Many of us have wrong beliefs about why we experience the things we do, about who is responsible for those things, whose fault they are, and even about what it is that is really happening.

Often, we find ourselves attributing the work of Satan to God and vise-versa, saying that what God is bringing about in our lives is the work of the devil. It is impossible to co-operate with the Holy Spirit if we do not have truthful beliefs about the circumstances we go through.

You can't judge circumstances as being "good" or not based on the standards the world uses. God's definition of good and bad and the world's definition of good and bad are not the same. God's will for Jesus involved pain and suffering. Yet God's will was good and perfect and the greatest good possible was brought out of something that most of us would have called bad.

The apostle Peter himself could not, at first, see God's hand in what Jesus was going to go through:

> "From that time on Jesus began to explain to his disciples that he must go to Jerusalem and suffer many things at the hands of the elders, chief priests and teachers of the law, and that he must be killed and on the third day be raised to life. Peter took him aside and began to rebuke him. "Never, Lord!" he said. "This shall never happen to you!" Jesus turned and said to Peter, "Get behind me, Satan! You are a stumbling block to me; you do not have in mind the things of God, but the things of men." (Matthew 16: 21-23)

Obviously, Peter misunderstood the circumstances. He thought it was wrong for Jesus to suffer and die. Remember how he cut the man's ear off in the garden when they came to take Jesus? Peter was prepared to fight back and to try to prevent it if he could (John 18: 10-11). His beliefs about the circumstances leading up to Jesus' death were, at this time, not correct or truthful. He was unable to cooperate with God in the advancement of the kingdom until his wrong thinking was corrected after Jesus' resurrection.

Many times we make the same mistakes. We make wrong judgments about the things that are happening to us or to others. Because we have preconceived notions of what we consider to be good, or right, or wrong, or fair, or unfair (often acquired from the world), we are unable to see the hand of God in our circumstances.

Job is a good example to look at. Everything was going very well for him at the beginning of the book. He was blessed, his kids were blessed, his stuff was blessed. He apparently was very careful to do everything in his power to ensure that the blessings on his life continued, even to the point of offering sacrifices for sins he thought his kids might have committed (Job 1: 4-5). Maybe he thought he was blessed because he was so careful to do what was right and that as long as he was careful to do what he thought was right God should continue to bless him. Then it all turned upside down.

His friends told him it was because of some sin of his, even though they couldn't quite put their finger on what the sin was. Most of the suffering Job experienced appears to be because he didn't know why all the bad things were happening to him. When God appeared to him out of the storm, at the end of the book, he still didn't know why. But he saw God revealed; he saw him as he really was. And he realized that God was still good in spite of everything he had gone through.

Job was vindicated because he continued to remain faithful to God even though it looked like God was unfair. If he had only looked on the outward appearance of his circumstances he would have cursed God, as his wife suggested, for deceiving him.

Besides having wrong beliefs about whether or not what is happening to us is good and fair or not, we also have wrong beliefs about who is responsible for why our lives are the way they are:

> "A man's own folly ruins his life, yet his heart rages against the Lord." (Proverbs 19: 3)

> "Do not be deceived: God cannot be mocked. A man reaps what he sows." (Galatians 6: 7)

When our life circumstances are pleasing often we pat ourselves on the back and tell ourselves what a good job we've done making everything work out so well (this is, itself, deceptive thinking). We like to take the credit when things are good. If our life circumstances are not pleasing often the first thing we do is look around for a scapegoat, someone or something to blame them on. When things are not going well we don't want to take the credit for that. People will blame their parents, their kids, their job, their spouse, their boss, the government, and especially God for why their lives are not what they want them to be.

We tell ourselves if others would just stop doing what they are doing or start doing what they are not doing, our lives would be better. You may not have power over other people to control the things they say and do, but you do have the ability to choose how you allow other people's choices and behavior to affect you.

Your circumstances must be judged in light of what you have sown by way of your own choices as well as in the light of God's kingdom purposes.

Look at the example of Adam. In Genesis 2, before Eve was created, God put him in the Garden of Eden and gave him the job of taking care of it. In verse 16 God said,

"You are free to eat from any tree in the garden; but you must not eat from the tree of the knowledge of good and evil, for when you eat of it you will surely die."

He said this to Adam before Eve appeared on the scene. She doesn't show up until verse 22. Maybe it was Adam's job to tell Eve about the tree.

In Genesis 3 the serpent comes up to Eve, not Adam, and

tempts her to eat from the tree. She tells the serpent what God has said about the tree. But then, the serpent gets her to question what she has heard.

Perhaps she thinks Adam may not have told her the whole story, or that God is hiding something from her. So she listens to what the serpent says. She takes the fruit and eats it and gives some to Adam who is right there with her while all this is going on (verse 6). There is no record of him speaking up to remind Eve about not eating the fruit. Yet later on, when they have been caught in sin, he seems to want to blame Eve even though the command to not eat of the tree was given to him before she was created.

He seems also to blame God when he says, "The woman you put here with me – she gave me some fruit from the tree and I ate it." Adam seems to be implying that ultimately the whole thing is God's fault because God put the woman there and if she had not been there, none of this would have happened.

It is important to make sure you are correctly "seeing" what is happening to you. Job was not allowed to see why he was being tested. He didn't get to see Satan come to God with the idea of ruining him to see if he would be faithful. But it is possible to discern, as much as you need to, what is happening and why.

Job discerned enough about the goodness of God to refuse to renounce him. God wants us to cooperate with him in his kingdom work. He wants us to make wise, informed choices in response to the things that happen to us in life. Better yet, he wants us to learn to make choices that determine where we go, and not just react to whatever circumstances come along.

You can apply this retroactively. You can look back to the

things you experienced before you were born again and judge them differently when you have a more truthful perception about why they happened and who was responsible. It's possible to change your beliefs and perception when you realize things didn't necessarily happen for the reason you thought they did and that the people you thought were responsible might not have been.

Many of your circumstances were created as you reaped what you and your past generations sowed. They didn't happen because God didn't love you or care about you.

Here are some examples of wrong beliefs about your circumstances:

1. It's not fair.

2. It's not my fault (this does not mean you must accept blame when you are innocent, it just means you should be careful to own up to the consequences of your own choices).

3. Everything bad always happens to me.

4. If I come out of my jail (the one I have in my mind) bad things will happen to me.

5. Nothing will ever change; things will never get better

6. I deserve better than this.

7. It's God's fault that bad things happen.

8. I won't reap what I sow.

9. If things are good, God is blessing me; if things are bad (or difficult) it must be the devil's fault.

10. Nothing good can possibly come out of what I am going through.

11. If I can't have what I want I can't be happy.

12. Right and wrong depend on the circumstances.

13. If it is God's will it will just happen all by itself.

14. Everything that happens is God's will.

Take a closer look:

1. Do you think you have correct, truthful beliefs about why your life is the way it is? How can you tell?

2. Can you discern God's hand in your circumstances? Give an example.

3. How does knowing God's hand is on your circumstances help you to deal with them?

4. Have you ever looked back on things that happened before you became a follower of Christ and seen them from a different perspective because of what you have learned of the truth? Explain.

5. What are some wrong beliefs you have had about things you have experienced? Give an example.

6. What does the Bible say about our circumstances and how we should respond to them? Write down some scriptures that talk about the circumstances of our lives and how we should respond to them below:

9

Ungodly Mindsets – Rejection, Resentment, Rebellion

> "Do not repay evil with evil or insult with insult. On the contrary, repay evil with blessing, because to this you were called so that you may inherit a blessing." (1 Peter 3:9)

Hopefully you have seen by now how important it is to have truthful beliefs if you are to navigate your way through life successfully and live in agreement with God. The devil has a vested interest in keeping you from knowing the truth that will set you free from slavery. One of the most successful strategies he has devised to keep people from knowing and worshipping God in spirit and truth is the rejection mindset.

We touched on this a little bit in a previous chapter and now want to look at it in more detail because so many people, to one degree or another, have been imprisoned by it. Remember we talked about how wrong beliefs create structures in the mind called strongholds. These strongholds are like prisons that keep people locked up away from truth, freedom, and the peace and security of God's love and presence. Freedom comes when the stronghold of lies is dismantled and replaced by a fortress of truth.

A mindset is different than a momentary perception. You can feel rejected by someone without it being a rejection mindset. A rejection mindset occurs when a person's whole life is lived from the perspective of believing they are unloved and unwanted.

To reject means to refuse to accept or consider, to refuse to admit, receive, or hear, to cast off or throw back (like you would throw a fish back if it wasn't big enough), or repulse. A person who has a rejection mindset believes they are unwanted, unloved, and feels cast off by others. They feel like the fish, which has been caught, examined, and then thrown back because it is not good enough, or is deficient in some way.

They feel like they don't fit in, that they are left out, and are conscious of a sense of shame, that there is something inherently wrong with them that keeps them from being accepted. Often the rejection mindset takes root early in life when love and acceptance are withheld (for whatever reason) by those whose responsibility is to feed love into the person's life (like the parents). Often the seeds of rejection are planted in a child before it is even born when the mother or father or both do not want the child.

God created us with the need to love and be loved. When that expectation is not met, when our love is not accepted and when we don't receive the love we expect to receive, rejection is experienced. If it is not dealt with the right way, a seed of rejection can be planted in a person's life. Future interactions with other people will be influenced by the presence of the seed of rejection.

Eventually rejection, if not processed correctly, will become rooted in the person's personality and become part of their "filter". The devil wants you to feel rejected. He knows if he can get you to believe you are not loved and not wanted you will be unable to receive God's love or give it to others. Since God is love and it is through the unconditional giving and receiving of love that his kingdom grows, it is easy to see how destructive a rejection mindset is in a believer's life.

People manifest different degrees of the rejection mindset. To some it is only a minor issue because for the most part they feel secure and accepted by the majority of the people in their lives. The rejection is confined to a few or certain people. There is enough giving and receiving of love from others to minimize the effects of rejection from these few people. In others, however, the rejection mindset is developed to the point where rejection is sensed all the time, everywhere, from everyone.

In this case rejection has become part of the person's filter. Other people's words and actions are interpreted as rejection even when that is not the intent. These people are literally shut off from experiencing love and acceptance because of the way they think. When love is offered, it is rejected because there is no trust. The person offering their love is suspected of ulterior motives and viewed with suspicion. The one with the rejection mindset has already decided no one can or will love them so any attempt by others to show love is rejected as being false or manipulative.

Rejection is real. We all experience it to one degree or another. That is not where the untruthful thinking comes in. A real experience of rejection can cause a person to begin to believe lies. They believe a lie when they believe they are unlovable and unacceptable by anyone because someone has rejected them.

There will always be people who do not like you. Not everyone is going to be your friend. But if you allow their behavior to cause you to believe lies about God and about the people who do want to like you and be your friend, then you have allowed a stronghold of rejection to be established in your mind.

Often rejection is the product of buying into the thinking of the world. Think about the women who feel unloved and unwanted because they don't measure up to the standards of beauty set out in popular culture. Think of the men who feel rejected because they don't measure up to the standards of "success" or masculinity held forth by the world.

When people don't meet the unrealistic (ungodly) standards that have been set they are often rejected by others who accept those standards as normal and right. Think of all the kids we have heard about in the news who took a gun to school and killed their classmates because they had been bullied and rejected. Why were they bullied? Often it was because they didn't fit in with what was considered normal or cool by their classmates.

The world tells us we have to be like everyone else or we won't be accepted or fit in. We have to live like the world says to live, want the stuff the world says we are supposed to want, and have the priorities the world says we should have, etc. Living as a follower of Jesus Christ is going to put us in conflict with the world. We have to stop believing that if we don't do things the way the world tells us to we won't be happy or fulfilled.

Rejection doesn't stop with a sense of being unwanted and not fitting in. Left unchecked, the root of rejection in a person's life will begin to grow and produce the fruit of resentment and rebellion. Resentment develops when a person responds to the sense of rejection with anger instead of forgiveness.

People who feel rejected will begin to resent those they

think are rejecting them. This resentment can manifest as outward hostility towards others or as withdrawing inwardly away from people and reality (or both). Outbursts of anger, attitudes of suspicion and mistrust, keeping people at a distance emotionally, and even physically are manifestations of resentment.

Resentment can also manifest as escaping into fantasy through games, movies, and T.V., and the development of depression. A lot of depression is really suppressed anger and resentment. Many people cannot resolve their anger because they believe it is wrong for them to feel angry in the first place, and to admit to the presence of anger in their life is to say they are a failure. A lot of Christians are like this.

Resentment can be directed inwardly where the person begins to reject their own self and hate what they are because they think there is something wrong with them that causes others to reject them. They believe others are rejecting what and who they are, not just their behavior. They will resent God because they hold him responsible for making them the way they are.

Resentment will manifest as unforgiveness and bitterness if left unchecked. These attitudes will, in turn, affect every other area of the person's life. God says our sins will not be forgiven if we do not forgive the sins of others (Matthew 18:21-35). A rejection mindset manifesting in resentment often blinds people to their own faults and sins while making them hypersensitive to the faults of others. They feel their resentment is justified and don't want to give it up. Because they don't forgive they end up being unable to sense God's presence and love.

Eventually, if it is not repented of, resentment will develop into full-blown rebellion. The person will rebel against everything and everyone that appears to them to be the source of their pain and misery. Because they see God as the primary problem (God made them the way they are) and because they are convinced he doesn't care about them, they will cast off restraint and self control and indulge in all kinds of destructive behavior.

Eating and drinking too much, overuse of artificial stimulants (drugs, tobacco), perverse and unclean sexual behavior, destruction of relationships through lying, deception, and irresponsibility, disregard for any and all types of authority, or complete withdrawal from interaction with other people (replacing it with excessive love for animals, fantasy and escapism) are examples of how this rebellion manifests.

This is the goal of the enemy. He leads people away from the protection, peace, and prosperity of living in relationship with God by getting them to believe a lie, and then draws them into the place of destruction. Because they don't believe God does love them or can love them they are cut off from the only remedy for their situation, which is God's love and forgiveness.

Rejection, resentment, and rebellion are often at the root of many of the destructive mindsets the Holy Spirit is trying to set us free from. Many of the ungodly attitudes we listed in earlier chapters have their roots in rejection mindsets.

The cure for the rejection mindset is to be convinced of God's unconditional love for you. When you finally believe he loves you and accepts you just as you are, and that you don't have to perform for or earn his love, you will be free to love and receive love unconditionally. When you realize his love is enough and you don't need to have everyone love you in order to have a sense of worth and be secure, you will be able to focus on loving others as God loves you instead of worrying about whether or not you are loved and accepted by them.

Coming out of agreement with the rejection mindset often takes a lot of time and persistent effort. It took me years. I struggled with rejection all my life. I was fearful of letting people get too close to me because I thought they would not like what they found. I tried to gain love by being what I thought people wanted me to be. I feared close personal interactions with others. I found my greatest peace in escaping into books and fantasy, daydreaming and imagination. There I could control my world and make it any way I wanted it to be.

God loved me enough to not let me stay in this place. I remember the day the revelation of God's unconditional love finally sank in. I finally really believed that he loved me just the way I was. It was the beginning of freedom. If I didn't need to perform for God anymore then I wasn't going to worry about having to perform for people.

God's love gave me enough of a sense of security to begin to take risks in relating to other people. I started to let my walls down. I found out that much of what I had feared of being rejected by others was a complete lie. And I began to discover the presence of demonic spirits in my life that had harassed me with lies for years.

The Holy Spirit started talking to me about all the attitudes and behaviors in my life that were rooted in rejection. Even silly things like getting angry because my husband didn't like the way I made pancakes. I thought by rejecting my cooking he was rejecting me personally. I thought when people didn't agree with me or see things the way I saw them it was because I wasn't good enough. I would fight with my husband trying to get him to admit I was right or to do things my way because that was the only way I felt worthwhile. What a relief to be able to lay it all down! What a relief to not have to fight and strive for acceptance and a sense of worth. And it all came from believing the truth.

Take a closer look:

1. Do you ever have the sense that you don't fit in or belong or that others are rejecting you?

2. Is this sense a major factor in your life? Does it influence how you relate to others and how you relate to God?

3. Are you able to handle rejection when it comes your way by forgiving, or do you find it hard to forgive and move on? Do you rehearse in your mind over and over the unkind things people do or say to you?

4. Are you secure in who you are? Do you like yourself? Do you believe others like you?

5. Are you secure in God's love for you? Or are you afraid his love might be withdrawn if you make a mistake or are not "good" enough?

6. Do you have resentment and unforgiveness in your life? If so, why? Towards whom?

7. Can you relate to people easily or do you find it stressful? If it is stressful, why?

8. Are you willing to let go of your anger and resentment towards those who have hurt you?

9. If you are, here is a prayer you can pray to get started along the road to peace and security in God:

Heavenly Father,

Thank you that you love me just the way I am. Thank you for what Jesus did on the cross so my sins can be forgiven.

Father I don't want to live any longer with burdens of rejection, resentment, bitterness, and unforgiveness. I want to be free to experience your love and sense your presence. Please forgive me for allowing wrong mindsets to be built in my mind. Forgive me for believing the lie that no one loves me or cares about me. I know you love me and care about me always.

Please forgive me for allowing resentment and bitterness to find a place in my heart. Forgive me for giving the enemy a seat of authority in my life and for allowing him to fill my mind with lies. I renounce the whole rejection, resentment, rebellion mindset.

I choose to believe that I am loved and accepted by you Father, and that is enough for me. I choose to believe that I don't have to be perfect or perform perfectly for you to love and accept me. So I will no longer demand that others be perfect or perform perfectly for me before I accept them and love them. I release to you all the people who have hurt or disappointed me in any way. I choose to forgive them now in Jesus name. Please cleanse me by the blood of Jesus from all bitterness and resentment. Give me grace to give up the lies that I am not loved or wanted or that I don't belong or fit in.

I choose from this day forward to believe the truth about myself and about you, Father. I will guard my mind and not allow untruthful thinking to have a place there. Satan, I release myself from your influence and control now in Jesus' name. I command all spirits of rejection, resentment, unforgiveness, and rebellion to leave in Jesus' name. Father, I will trust you to reveal to me the truth as I read your word and listen to your Spirit. Thank you for making me whole and healing my broken heart and spirit. I love you Lord and I know you love me.

In Jesus' name, amen.

10

Demonic Interference
in the Mind

"For our struggle is not against flesh and blood..." (Ephesians 6:12)

So far we have talked about how beliefs are acquired and how they develop to form a system through which we process life with all its various experiences. We have talked about how, before we are born again and receive the Holy Spirit (whose job is to re-acquaint us with truth), our belief systems are built on lies and deception. We have seen how a belief system that is built of lies and deception becomes a jail in the mind where a person is trapped in ungodly thinking and cannot realize the fullness of God's blessing and freedom.

This jail of ungodly, untruthful beliefs locks a person away from fulfilling their purpose in the kingdom. There is another element to this jail that we want to talk about now. It is the presence of demonic spirits in the mind.

Every jail I have ever seen has guards whose job is to keep the prisoners from escaping. If someone tries to break out of the jail the guards will go after them, round them up, and shove them back into their cell. The jails we have in our minds have guards too.

These guards are demon spirits whose job is keeping you from getting out of your jail. Many people do not realize that where there are lies and deception, there is sure to be the presence of demons. Demons are attracted to lies because that is their nature: they are liars and deceivers. That is how they gain control over a person, through lies and deception. Remember, our beliefs were formed in a world system based in lies and deception before we came to Christ. These demon jailers use their power and influence to keep us from recognizing and coming into agreement with God's truth.

Sin is the open door through which demons gain access into a person's life. All sin starts in the mind:

> "When tempted, no one should say, "God is tempting me." For God cannot be tempted by evil, nor does he temp anyone; but each person is tempted when they are dragged away by their own evil desire and enticed. Then, after desire has conceived, it gives birth to sin, and sin, when it is full-grown, gives birth to death." (James 1: 13-15)

First there is temptation in some form or other that registers in the mind. Then there is the contemplation of that temptation, whether or not it will be acted on. Finally, there is the choice made to either give in to the temptation or reject it.

Temptations from the enemy usually come disguised in some way. They are deceiving. Eve gave in to the temptation to eat the fruit because she was deceived and believed a lie about God.

When we believe lies and then begin to make choices that are motivated by that lie it is sin. God gives us permission to believe what is true. We, as his kingdom covenant people, are not allowed to believe whatever we want. We are allowed to believe his word, which is truth. So when we believe a lie from the enemy, and begin to act on it, it's sin.

At some point, as sin is indulged over and over again, access is made for demon spirits to gain entrance to our bodies and minds. Lies that are believed and acted on over time will provide demons with access. Nobody knows exactly where the line is between just believing something that isn't true and where a demon shows up and uses that belief to merge its evil nature and person with our own.

Houseguest

If you invited someone to your house, to come in and sit down and share a meal with you, we would say you were entertaining them. We could say you found your guest to be agreeable in some way. If you didn't you would probably show them the door and not invite them back again or you would not have invited them in the first place.

If the presence of your guest was agreeable, you could invite them to stay with you for a while. Their presence in your home would have an influence on how you lived your life. When thoughts come to our minds and we ponder them and think about them a lot, we call it entertaining an idea or thought. Revelation 3: 20 says:

> "Here I am! I stand at the door and knock. If anyone hears my voice and opens the door, I will come in and eat with him, and he with me."

Jesus wants us to entertain him. He wants us to invite him in via believing his truth and give him a place to sit down (a place of authority) in our lives so we can have continuous fellowship with him.

It is possible to entertain the devil the same way. Let's say Satan shows up at the door of your mind with a thought or idea. He knocks on the door. If you open the door, and invite him and his idea or thought to come in and sit down with you, you are entertaining him. If, after looking over his idea or thought for a while as you engage him in conversation, you allow him to stay, you are giving him a place of influence and control in your life.

Satan, being who he is, will shortly invite a lot of his friends to come join him. Pretty soon your house is going to be filled with him and his friends, each one bringing another thought or idea with them. Together, all these ideas and thoughts will create a jail and Satan and his friends will be more than happy to guard the jail to make sure you don't get out.

Agreement with the devil is when you invite him in, entertain him and his thoughts and then let him stay. Each lie that you entertain and accept gives the enemy a greater seat of control, influence, and authority over your life. This is how demons gain entrance and how demonic strongholds (jails) are built in your mind. Demons reinforce ungodly, untruthful thinking and beliefs by manipulating perceptions and emotions, and blind people to the truth.

A person who attempts to begin the process of renewing their mind will often find they run right into resistance from demons that fight back against any attempts made to dislodge them. They want you to stay in your jail and seek to become part of the filter through which you process life.

When we talk about the power of a demon spirit to distort our perception we are talking about something that is very real. The presence of demons can literally keep you from being able to see what is right in front of you. Demonic power and influence can pervert and distort the things you see and hear so you interpret them the wrong way. Let's look at the example of the Gadarene demoniac:

> "When Jesus got out of the boat, a man with an evil spirit came from the tombs to meet him. This man lived in the tombs, and no one could bind him anymore, not even with a chain. For he had often been chained hand and foot, but he tore the chains apart and broke the irons on his feet. No one was strong enough to subdue him. Night and day among the tombs and in the hills he would cry out and cut himself with stones." (Mark 5: 2-5)

Today we would say this man was mentally ill. The demons inhabiting his mind and body destroyed his ability to live in the real world as a sound, rational human being. He couldn't think straight and his tormented mind was not working right because the demons were interfering with his perception and thought processes. This interference was very real and manifested in the symptoms of mental illness.

> "Those tending the pigs ran off and reported this (the casting out of the demons) in the town and countryside, and the people went out to see what had happened. When they came to Jesus, they saw the man who had been possessed by the legion of demons, sitting there, dressed and in his right mind. . ." (Mark 5: 14-15)

Once he got rid of the demons, the man was restored to a right, sound mind. This is an extreme example to be sure, although it is common enough in some parts of the world. The difference between this man and many of us is only a matter of degree. The demon spirits inhabiting his mind were able to interfere with his thought processes to keep him from living a normal, healthy, functional life.

It would have been pointless for Jesus to try to share the gospel with this man or impart to him truth and revelation as long as the demons were there. They would only have messed it up and perverted it in his mind or kept him from recognizing it for what it was.

> "The god of this age has blinded the minds of unbelievers so that they cannot see the light of the gospel of the glory of Christ, who is the image of God." (2 Corinthians 4: 4)

This is real blindness, not just a metaphor. These people are blinded to the truth. The word unbeliever doesn't just mean unsaved people. An unbeliever is one who does not believe. What is it they don't believe? The truth. Wherever there is the absence of truth there is blindness. Wherever there is entrenched blindness you will find the presence of demonic spirits.

Have you ever talked to someone and presented them with facts that were undeniable only to have it seem like they just bounced off the person? Have you ever talked to people where it seemed like you were talking to a wall, and what you were saying was just not getting through? People have blind spots in their thinking and perception that keep them from seeing what they need to see. And I think many of us would be surprised if the Lord opened our eyes into the spiritual realm and showed us how much of this blindness is caused by the presence of demon spirits.

I know I was surprised. The presence of demonic powers in my mind was made very real to me. Generational patterns of sin, especially occult sin, had allowed curses to be enforced against my family and me. Much of this was manifested as mental oppression and torment in the mind.

These demons of mental oppression and torment had lain dormant in my life until the right time came for them to manifest their presence. It was at a moment of weakness and stress when they chose to make their presence known. Out of the blue my life changed overnight as spirits of fear, rejection, curses of insanity and mental oppression began to manifest. I started having thoughts of suicide and was overwhelmed with fear. I started having panic attacks that got so bad I didn't want to leave the house. I actually quit driving for four years because I was afraid of having a panic attack while driving and getting into a wreck.

All of a sudden I could see up close and personal the influences that had tried to control my thinking and beliefs for years. Only now they were magnified to a whole new level. A lot of things became clear to me as I realized how many of the things I had struggled with had been caused by the presence of demon spirits oppressing my mind.

The demonic presence is like a veil over the mind that causes the input coming in to be distorted, perverted, or even completely hidden. I have met a lot of Christians who were blinded in their minds to some degree or who had their perception and ability to see truth compromised and distorted by the presence of demons.

Remember, it is not a matter of ownership. We belong to Christ and are his redeemed people. But if his redeemed people are deceived and believe a lie and begin to act on that lie, the possibility of a demon gaining a seat of control and influence in their life is just as real as it is for unbelievers. It is a matter of agreement.

Agreement with the enemy's lies gives him a place of control and influence in your life plain and simple. Such agreement opens the door to invasion by demon spirits whose presence will blind the mind and distort the perception in order to keep the person bound up in a place of barrenness and unfruitfulness.

"For although they knew God, they neither glorified him as God nor gave thanks to him, but their thinking became futile and their foolish hearts were darkened." (Romans 1: 21)

"They exchanged the truth of God for a lie, and worshiped and served created things rather than the Creator – who is forever praised. Amen." (Romans 1: 25)

Demonic blindness comes when there is departure from the truth. It comes through the generations as lies are passed down through families, religions, cultures, or other associations. You must understand that renewing the mind can involve more than adopting new beliefs. It may require you to remove the guards of the jail before the person locked inside can get out.

Take a closer look:

1. Have you ever seen or dealt with a person who seemed to have something blocking their mind so they couldn't see things that were very obvious?

2. How does agreement give demons access into our lives?

3. Are there any areas of your thinking that you think might be influenced by demons? What are they?

4. What makes you think so?

11

Evidence of the Presence of Demons in the Mind

"Thus, by their fruit you will recognize them."
(Matthew 7:20)

Demons leave signs that indicate they are present. If you were out in the woods you might see animal tracks. You might be able to tell what kind of animal left the track because each animal has distinct footprints. It is the same with demons. They leave "footprints" that tell you they are there and what kind of demon they are. A mind that is under the influence or control of demons will show symptoms.

My symptoms were varied. It felt like there was something trying to interfere with and inject itself into my mind against my will. Thoughts and pictures would come into my mind without me having willed them, but it still felt like it was me thinking them. I felt like there was some intelligent force that was trying to manipulate my perception and present the world to me so I would see it in a certain way. I had to fight against the influences continually and willfully reject the beliefs (often along with the emotions those beliefs stirred up) they were trying to enforce. I felt like I was a spy behind enemy lines watching and observing in my own life how the demonic

95

powers worked to drive someone crazy.

Most of the symptoms of the presence of demons in the mind manifest as disturbances in the thoughts. Some of these are listed below:

1. A mind that goes "blank". This does not mean every lapse of memory is caused by a demon. It just means when a person experiences it often, and there is no physical reason for it, and there are other symptoms of disturbances in the thoughts, it would be wise to consider the presence of demonic influences.

2. Voices, chattering, talking in the mind; especially voices that are uncontrollable. These voices can be in the first person where it seems like you yourself are thinking the thoughts.

3. Pictures flashing in the mind involuntarily. These can be either "nice" pictures or evil ones. (Not to be confused with prophetic vision.)

4. Mental confusion, inability to follow a train of thought, chronic difficulty in making decisions.

5. Chronic double-mindedness

6. A very passive mind, where the effort to think feels like wading through molasses.

7. A mind that won't shut off. Thoughts that are repeated endlessly, especially those that result in obsessive, compulsive behavior.

8. Bondages and addictions to fantasy and escapism, pornography, daydreaming, or drug use. This can be

through movies, television, books, games, recreational drugs or whatever, where the result is the inability to live in the real world or to give up the source.

9. The presence in the generations of lies and deception, especially cultural or religious deception. This would be something like generational mindsets of prejudice and victimization, cultural mindsets that demean women, or false religious teachings such as Jehovah's Witnesses, Mormonism, Buddhism, or denominational thinking that denies obvious truths of scripture, etc.

10. Frequent headaches, especially migraines.

11. Chronic depression and negativity. The feeling that a black cloud follows you wherever you go. Constant negative, critical, cynical thinking.

12. Pressure on the mind. This is a physical symptom; you can feel it, like having your brain in a vise.

13. Frequent nightmares and bad dreams.

14. The uneasy sensation that your mind does not seem to be working right.

15. The injection of thoughts, pictures, emotions, and feelings, against the person's will or desire.

16. Ungodly thought responses to circumstances or thought responses that are out of proportion to what has been experienced. An example of this would be an inundation of angry thoughts when someone does something you don't like. Only the level of anger would be out of proportion to what actually happened.

17. Any symptoms of mental illness such as schizophrenia, paranoia and paranoid delusions, manic depression, hearing audible voices or seeing apparitions.

If such disturbances are left unchecked they can result in what we call distortion of the mind. The presence of demons will cause the person's perception to be warped. Eventually this perversion of their perception will cause a distortion in the mind where the person begins to lose touch with reality and truth. The demons prevent them from correctly perceiving the world and their experiences and they begin to accept these distortions as the truth. If the person continues on the path, the end result can be the destruction of rational thought processes.

I personally believe that a lot of what we call mental illnesses and "syndromes" today are the result of demonic interference in the mind that has resulted from agreement with lies and deception, either in the present or past generations (or both). Sin and disobedience through the believing of lies and rejecting of truth open the doors (Romans 1: 18-32).

I believe my own experience in this area was the result of generational influences that pushed me into behaviors and attitudes that opened the door to demonic invasion in my mind. I believe the curses of insanity in my family were the result, at least in part, of occult sin. The enemy used it all to try to drive me over the edge into mental illness. Only the presence of the Holy Spirit, the Spirit of Truth, in my life kept me from falling victim to the enemy's plans.

"However, if you do not obey the Lord your God and do not carefully follow all his commands and decrees I am giving you today, all these curses will come on you and overtake you: The Lord will afflict you with madness, blindness and confusion of mind. At midday you will grope about like a blind person in the dark." (Deuteronomy 28: 15, 28-29)

Demons will use their power to pervert a person's thought processes in order to drive them to certain kinds of thinking, belief, and behavior. Demons are the original propaganda artists. They will blind a person to what he or she needs to see and cause the input from life experiences to be selectively presented in order to reinforce the ungodly mindset.

It's like people talking about the "good old days". Memory is selective. We tend to remember things the way we want to remember them and often forget over time the way things actually were. Demons promote this kind of selective memory so that our worldview and perspective on life are not truthful. The goal is to keep us from seeing and coming into agreement with truth.

We can look at the example of Saul in the Old Testament. He was the anointed king of Israel. But over time, as he was careless about obeying God (1 Samuel 15), and began to harbor jealousy and resentment towards David (1 Samuel 18) an evil spirit came upon him and drove him to violent behavior. Eventually he ended up unable to hear the voice of God, tormented with paranoid thoughts. He murdered the priests of God because he thought they were against him (1 Samuel 22) and went to consult a witch to find out what he was to do (1 Samuel 28). His habitual sin gave place to demon spirits to torment him. As he refused to repent, he descended further and further into paranoid thinking and behavior.

Take a closer look:

1. After looking at the list above, which, if any, of these

symptoms have you experienced?

2. Is there evidence in your family line of entrenched ungodly thinking? We mean things that are passed down through the generations. Explain.

3. Have you ever had the experience of feeling like something in your mind was trying to force itself on you against your will either through thoughts, feelings, or pictures in your head?

4. Can you say your mind is at peace and rest most of the time?

5. Have you ever felt like something was fighting back when you attempted to fill your mind with truth? Explain.

6. What other symptoms have you experienced that may not be on the list but you think might be the result of demonic influences in your mind?

12

Mental Illness

> "God has not given us a spirit of fear, but of
> power and of love and of a sound mind." (2
> Timothy 1:7 NKJV)

Mental illness has been with us throughout the ages. It has
no regard for age, race, gender, or socio-economic status. There
are mentally ill people who are rich and who are poor, who are
young and who are old, male and female alike. Doctors and
psychiatrists for the most part do not know what causes mental
illness. They can recognize the symptoms and often detect
physiological changes in the body that seem to accompany
some mental illness. This leads them to suspect that mental
illness is physical in nature.

Most of the treatment prescribed for mental illness today
involves the use of pills and various medications, counseling, or
a combination of them both, or even electric shock therapy
where the idea is to stimulate the neural transmitters in the
brain that are supposedly causing mental illness because they
are not working right.

Some people are helped with these approaches. Insanity
can be caused by toxic substances, such as mercury that
accumulate in the fatty tissue of the brain. Mental illnesses can

be caused by emotional trauma that must be worked through. For a lot of people, though, these treatments produce marginal results if any at all.

In the past, people who were mentally ill were often confined to an institution, especially if their symptoms were severe. Mentally ill people many times become the object of abuse by others in their family. The stress of dealing with mental illness can be so overwhelming people just lose patience because they are so frustrated.

I believe God is our source of healing from mental illness just as he is for all other kinds of sickness and disease. There is mental illness that is spiritual in nature that does not respond to natural treatment approaches. Deuteronomy 28: 1-14 gives us a picture of God's idea of "normal" for his people. It talks about blessing and wholeness and soundness as our right state of being. This is the way we are supposed to live. Anything else is not normal.

It is sad to say but most people find their "normal" in the rest of the chapter to one degree or another. Verse 15 and following talk about the opposite of blessing, which is cursing. Blessing is the result of obedience; cursing is the result of disobedience. It is interesting to read what some of the symptoms of cursing are. They include wasting diseases and illnesses that have no cure (verse 21-22, 27). It also talks about mental problems in verse 28, namely, madness, confusion of mind, and blindness. Mental illness is not what God wants for his people. Directly or indirectly, sin and disobedience are the cause of all the issues we struggle with. I believe a lot of mental illness has its roots there too.

How do we define mental illness? It appears to result when the mind is placed under sustained stress loads that it was not designed to handle. After a while of being under this kind of stress, it just quits, like a circuit that blows out because too much current is coming through.

God created mankind to live within certain boundaries. There are boundaries for our behavior, our choices, our relationships, and our thinking and beliefs. For example, our bodies were designed to function well under certain conditions. They require rest, the right kind of healthy food, a certain amount of exercise, and will cease to function well (or at all) if they are subjected to abuse in these areas.

Go ahead and eat nothing but junk food for a whole year and see what kind of condition you find yourself in at the end of it. Or, don't exercise, get less sleep than you need, and watch what happens to your body. Why should we think our minds are any different? If they are subjected to stress levels they are not designed to handle we shouldn't be surprised if they stop functioning.

My own issues with mental oppression were the result of entrenched ungodly thinking combined with generational influences rooted in occult practices. The stresses created from ungodly, untruthful mindsets were magnified by demonic spirits who tried to use them to drive me over the edge.

Constant chatter in my head, tormenting demonic dreams that seemed like they were really happening, together with the feeling that something was playing with my mind were some of the symptoms I experienced. Then there were the panic attacks. I was a mess. What was kind of weird was the way the things in my mind seemed to know that I knew what they were. I knew they were demons and they knew that I knew.

Roots of mental illness

A lot of mental illness is the result of the influence of generational curses that are triggered by some kind of stress. There are people who are suffering from curses of insanity that have roots way back in their generations. All that is needed to release the symptoms of mental illness is stress of some kind that is either self-imposed or imposed by the behaviors of others, or imposed by demons (or a combination of some or all of the above).

A lot of this stress can come from living outside the boundaries God has established. Messing with the occult, sexual sin, the use of drugs, alcohol, and fantasy to escape from real life, lying and deception, uncontrolled emotional outbursts etc. can all provide plenty of stresses that God never intended us to have to deal with. Demons often remain dormant in a person's life until the right moment comes along when they choose to manifest their presence. They wait until they see a moment of weakness and then exploit it. Ungodly stress loads provide that moment.

A lot of mental illness works like this. It seems like, suddenly, overnight, or over a short period of time, a person goes from being sound in their mind and personality to falling apart. I know of two different women whose problems with mental illness and torment started when they left home to live on their own. The demons causing the mental illness used the stresses of fear (such as fear of failure, or fear of the unknown, or fear of being rejected by people), insecurity and anxiety and blew everything out of proportion in their minds.

As time went on, the pressure from overload in the mind that was coming from constant demonic harassment caused them to short-circuit and have what we call a nervous breakdown. Normally, the experience of leaving home can certainly be stressful. It was the presence in the person's life of demonic interference and generational curses however, that caused the stresses to become magnified to the point they became unbearable.

Demons have power to manipulate the mind. They can distort and pervert the information and input that come into our minds from our five senses. They can cause us to see and hear things that are not there and to not see and hear things that are there. They can distort perception to the point where everything looks like it is being reflected in a carnival mirror. A person subjected to this kind of demonic oppression can feel like they are losing their mind.

In Chapter 7 we used the example of the Gadarene demoniac. It was the presence in him of all those demons that overloaded his mind to the point he no longer behaved like a rational human being.

The demonic interference that can lead to mental illness comes from several sources. It comes from generational curses, especially curses from the sin of occult practices. When people participate in such things as the Ouija board, tarot cards, and séances, when they attempt to gain ungodly access into the spirit realm for the purposes of gaining information and control, mental illness and insanity are often the result.

Human beings are not capable in themselves of dealing with the stress that comes from ungodly contact with the spirit world. The only contact with the spirit realm we are supposed to have is what we are given by God and allowed to exercise under his Lordship and with his permission. Anything else will result in levels of stress on the mind that will cause it to eventually collapse. People who are involved in occult practices suffer very high levels of mental illness and breakdown.

Demonic interference in the mind that results in mental illness and insanity can come from your own sins that are not repented of. Sin of any kind gives the enemy an open door of opportunity to infiltrate your mind and body. You may not always experience the full manifestation of this infiltration right away. The enemy will allow you to be like the frog in the pot. The water in the pot where the frog was placed was heated up so gradually the frog never noticed until he was too weak and relaxed to jump out. At the right moment of perceived weakness demons will spring their trap.

People are often too weak to resist the enemy when the sudden realization of his presence in their lives blows up in their face. They have been too used to giving in to his more subtle manipulation and pressure and there is no way they can withstand a full, frontal assault. Strongholds of fear, anger, bitterness, hatred (especially of God's people - anti-Semitism) sexual perversion, or whatever will attempt to overwhelm a person in their mind and emotions and will distort their perception until they no longer operate in a sound, rational, godly, truthful mind.

Mental illness can also come from the development of ungodly, untruthful beliefs and mindsets that a person refuses to give up. As we said earlier in this book, agreement with the lies of the enemy gives him a place of influence and seat of authority in our lives. If a person still continues to cling to lies and deception even after they have been shown the truth, demonic strongholds will eventually prevent the person from being able to function in a normal (godly is normal as far as we are concerned) manner. The Bible talks about what happens to those who trade truth for lies (Romans 1: 21, 25, 28):

> "For although they knew God, they neither glorified him as God nor gave thanks to him, but their thinking became futile and their foolish

hearts (minds) were darkened."

"They exchanged the truth about God for a lie, and worshiped and served created things rather than the Creator - who is forever praised. Amen."

"Furthermore, just as they did not think it worthwhile to retain the knowledge of God, so God gave them over to a depraved mind, so that they do what ought not be done."

Take the example of a mother who is grieving over the loss of a child. Grief is a normal reaction to the death of a loved one up to a certain point. However, when a mother insists on leaving her child's room untouched, like a shrine (even though the child died twenty years ago), when she refuses to give love and attention to her husband and other children because she is devoting all of it to her deceased child, or when the rest of the family takes a back seat to the memory of the lost child there is danger that the mother is going to end up deceived if she doesn't allow the Lord to heal her of her grief.

She may go further and attempt to contact her lost child through a medium in a séance or begin to show anger towards those who don't reverence the memory of the child like she does. There have been cases where demons begin to manifest to people who are trapped in excessive grief over a lost loved one, disguised as that loved one.

This mother may not realize it but her mental perspective is becoming warped and distorted because she is departing from the truth with regard to how she is processing the loss of her child. Remember, mental illness is the result of stresses on the mind that it was not designed to deal with. God has a right way for us to handle the issues and traumas that happen as a part of life on this earth. If we don't do it his way, we can't expect to remain healthy and whole and sound.

Jesus is the healer of the mind

Mental illness is tricky to deal with. The presence of demons in the person's mind can make attempts at helping them difficult. Each case is unique. The Holy Spirit alone can direct a person's recovery from mental illness. It can be supernatural, as the Gadarene demoniac's was. Or it may be a process that takes place over time as untruthful thinking and beliefs are confronted and given up and demons are cast out. One thing I do know. It is not impossible.

We must not be afraid to confront the issue of mental illness. Why do we think God is willing and able to heal physical illness but then pack off all cases of mental illness to the worldly psychologist or psychiatrist? Why are we afraid to tackle the problem of mental illness? God created the mind. He is the best healer of the mind.

I am not a mental health professional. I do know what worked in my own life and has helped other people. Mental oppression can be overcome. It takes dedication and perseverance. It takes commitment to the truth of God's word. The process cannot be rushed or pushed.

A person who needs help in this area must be convinced that God is able and willing to deliver and heal (I am assuming they are cognizant enough to participate in the healing process). There must be willingness to change and to give up mindsets and beliefs that are untruthful and ungodly. There must be willingness to commit to the word of God as the pattern of wholeness and truth. There must be willingness to come out of agreement with all thinking and behavior that results from demonic influence.

The demons involved must be cast out and the person must learn to keep them out. It is a big job. God is big enough to do it. Coming out of mental illness requires support from other people who will be able help keep the person seeking healing on the right path and who can help point out that path to them when they can't see it. A person struggling with mental illness needs people who will tell them the truth in love, and who will stand by them as a model of what a sound mind looks like.

My own path to freedom from mental oppression has taken a long time. Much longer, in fact, than I thought it would when I first began to struggle with it. I believe there are two primary principles that helped me get the victory in my situation. The first is I was committed to the truth of the word of God. I knew what I was dealing with was not caused by a chemical imbalance. I don't know how but I just knew it was demonic.

I knew the only remedy for my situation was God and his word. I grabbed onto the word and refused to let go no matter what my feelings or the demons were trying to tell me. I refused to accept anything that was contrary to what God said. When spirits of fear were telling me I would end up in a mental institution, I refused to believe it. When they tried to tell me I would never get better, I refused to believe it. When they tried to tell me God didn't love me because if he did why would he let something like this happen, I refused to believe it. I knew somehow that I had to hang on to the truth with an iron grip and be vehement in casting down every thought, feeling, emotion, symptom, or whatever that exalted itself against the knowledge of God.

Second, I knew I had to keep my attitude right. If I gave in to thoughts of resentment, or self-pity, or got angry with God for letting these things happen to me I knew I was finished. I had to count it all joy; I had to trust that tomorrow would be a better day, and that, eventually the day would come when I would be free.

That better day came when we got in touch with a man who knew something about dealing with demons. I had been prayed for by other people with no results. This man knew what he was doing. I remember what it felt like the first time one of those spirits left me. It was pretty dramatic. I could actually feel a dark oppressive thing lift off me and go. The first ones to be dealt with were the spirits of fear. When they left, things were different. And I knew I could no longer allow fear to control me or direct my life.

Once they were gone I had to keep them out. I also knew if we could get rid of one devil then we could get rid of all of them. Hope sprang up in me for the first time in a long time. The fight was far from over but my path was set and I never looked back. I gained freedom as the nature of the demonic spirits I was dealing with was revealed and I came out of agreement with the mindsets, behaviors and attitudes that kept me in bondage to them. I won't say it was easy. It was hard. It took a long time. I kept after it because I felt I didn't have a choice. The alternative (giving up or giving in, or a life spent dependent on strong, mind-altering drugs) was not even worth considering.

I remember watching my husband leave on a business trip one time. And I remember thinking to myself, "That is going to be me some day. Some day I am going to be able go places again like that without having to deal with all the demonic junk." God has been faithful. I have gained my freedom by degrees over the years. The Holy Spirit has shown me what I am fighting with and the ungodly mindsets I have needed to come out of agreement with in order to gain my freedom. I don't have panic attacks any more. I don't have the torment in my mind that I had for years. God's word has worked. The truth has set me free.

I wish there were some kind of formula that would just work for everyone who struggles with mental oppression. There isn't. Love, faith, trust, and obedience are what works. For those who are not in a position to help themselves, we must get to a place of power and authority in the kingdom where we can step in and see them released from bondage.

Take a closer look:

1. Do you know anyone who suffers from mental oppression?

2. Have you ever or do you now suffer from mental illness yourself?

3. Have you ever suspected that the source of your mental illness or that of the people you know might be spiritual rather than physical? If so, why do you think so?

4. Do you know anyone who can help you understand the source of your mental illness or that of the people you know and how to deal with it?

5. If you think you might be helped, ask the Lord to connect you with someone who can walk with you and counsel you on your journey back to wholeness.

13

The Restoration Process

"You were taught, with regard to your former way of life, to put off your old self, which is being corrupted by its deceitful desires; to be made new in the attitude of your minds; and to put on the new self, created to be like God in true righteousness and holiness." (Ephesians 4: 22-24)

So far we have looked at how mindsets are developed and how demons exploit sin and ungodly thinking to lock people up in jails in their minds. Now we come to the good part. The great news is you don't have to stay this way. God has provided you with the way to get out of jail. Like you used to do when you played Monopoly and drew the "get out of jail free" card from the deck. He has essentially slipped you a file so you can cut through the bars that keep you imprisoned.

We want to talk now about the process of renewal that will set us free in our minds and build a place of protection from the enemy's lies and deception. In the chapter where we discussed tearing down and building up, we began to touch upon the process through which renewing of the mind is achieved. We want to examine this process further in this chapter and look at the specific steps involved in renewing our minds. You need to remember that putting on the "new self" is something you do, not something someone else does for you. You have to choose to put off the old, to change your attitude, and to put on the new.

Admit the need

In order for your mind to be renewed several things have to happen. First, there must come the personal realization that there is a need for your own mind to be renewed. We must grasp the fact that much of our thinking and belief is not truthful and not kingdom oriented. Only when we realize there is a problem will we be motivated to begin and stick with the process of renewal.

After reading this far in this book you hopefully have an idea of whether or not there is a need to renew your own mind. However, agreeing with the statements in this book is not the same as actually experiencing renewing of the mind. There are a lot of Christians who think understanding these things and intellectually believing them to be true is the same as having a renewed mind.

Many of us have made the mistake of compartmentalizing our thinking without even realizing it. On Sunday we switch to Christian mode while we are in church and say amen to the things we hear. Monday through Saturday (or whatever) we switch to living-in-the-world mode and often the things we were taught on Sunday are forgotten and never get put into practice.

It is important you don't let this happen. The things you learn about renewing your mind must be lived out and applied on a day-to-day basis consistently in order for your mind to be truly renewed. Stop here for a moment and think. Allow the

Holy Spirit to speak to you about the need to renew your own mind. If you sense the twinge of conviction, that there is a need for renewal in your own thinking and beliefs, write down below your own personal statement to the Lord.

Acknowledge to him that you realize you need to have your mind renewed. Ask him to begin to show you the areas in your thinking and beliefs that need to be changed. Ask him to guide and direct your steps through the renewal process. Commit yourself to allowing the Holy Spirit to change your thinking and to renew your mind in truth. Sign your name and date it. (If there is not enough room in the space provided, get another piece of paper.)

My commitment to renew my mind:

_____

_____

_____

_____

_____

Signed by: Date:

_____   _____

Your stuff

The next step in the renewal process is to identify the mindsets and beliefs you have that are not truthful, and not in agreement with God's kingdom ways. This will probably happen over time, especially as you commit to spend time regularly in your Bible (where you will find lots of truth). The Holy Spirit will not make you bite off more than you can chew. It takes time to be able to see where your thinking and beliefs are wrong. Sometimes you need other people to help you see things you can't discern on your own. This is where you need to be humble.

It's hard hearing people point out where you are wrong. Pride makes it hard to admit fault of any kind. Often people respond to someone telling them stuff about themselves that they don't want to hear by pointing out the other person's flaws and shortcomings. Neither response gets you where you want to go.

> "Whoever loves discipline loves knowledge,
> but whoever hates correction is stupid."
> (Pro. 12: 1)

> "Whoever disregards discipline comes to
> poverty and shame, but whoever heeds
> correction is honored."
> (Pro. 13: 18)

Your decision to renew your mind has nothing to do with whether or not anyone else wants to renew theirs. You can't say, "Well, I'll admit where I'm wrong if you admit where you are." You have to want to change your life bad enough to deal with your stuff even if no one else wants to deal with theirs. You have nothing to lose and much to gain by humbly considering the input from other people.

Take some time to pray and ask the Holy Spirit to point out the mindsets and beliefs in your own life that need to be changed. Ask him to show you the beliefs and mindsets about God, about yourself, about other people, and about your life and circumstances that he wants to address.

Prayer:

Father God,

Thank you for making a way for me to come out of darkness so I can walk in the light of truth. Thank you that your love for me is steadfast and unchanging. I acknowledge right now that you, Jesus, are Lord of my life and that my mind and everything in it belongs to you. I want to glorify you in every aspect of my life and I want to be free from the lies and deception of the world so I can walk with you, love, and worship you in truth.

Holy Spirit, please show me where lies and deception have become part of my "filter". Please begin the process of making me aware of where my mindsets and beliefs are not truthful. Give me grace to see what I have not yet been able to see. Help me correctly identify the roots of these beliefs and mindsets so I can deal with them effectively and be set free to believe the truth. Thank you for what you are going to do in my life as my mind is renewed.

In Jesus name, amen.

Write down the things the Holy Spirit shows you:

1. Wrong beliefs about God:

_____

_____

_____

_____

_____

_____

2. Wrong beliefs about myself:

_____

_____

_____

_____

_____

3. Wrong beliefs about other people:

_____

_____

_____

_____

_____

4. Wrong beliefs about my life and circumstances:

_____

_____

_____

_____

_____

_____

Repent

As the Holy Spirit shows you where your thinking is wrong you need to repent of wrong, ungodly, untruthful beliefs and of the lies you have accepted as truth. Name these wrong beliefs as specifically as possible.

For example, if you allowed yourself to believe you are stupid and worthless because you were told that by your parents, or friends, or whoever, you need to repent of believing that lie. You know this is a lie because God's word says you are not worthless and that he didn't make you stupid. You then forgive the people whose words helped warp your sense of worth and identity.

To repent means to turn away from. As truth is revealed you must make the choice to turn away from lies and refuse to believe them any longer.

Prayer:

Father God,

Thank you for your love for me. Thank you for making a way for me to be free in my mind by knowing the truth. Thank you for giving me the Spirit of Truth so I can know what truth is. Forgive me Lord for believing lies about myself, about you, about other people, and about my life and circumstances. Forgive me for the choices I made to agree with things that were not truthful (state any specific beliefs the Holy Spirit shows you). I repent, and from today forward I will make new choices to believe the truth as you reveal it to me.

I forgive those whose influence promoted the belief of lies and wrong thinking. I forgive them and release myself from their words in Jesus' name. I renounce all ungodly, untruthful beliefs about myself (name any specific ones the Holy Spirit shows you), about you, God (name the ones the Holy Spirit shows you), about other people (name the person or persons and the belief), and about my life and circumstances (name the ones the Holy Spirit shows you). I turn from these beliefs and commit to replacing them with the truth. I will trust the Holy Spirit to lead me and guide me into all truth.

In Jesus' name, amen.

Bringing down the walls

This brings you to the next step which is found in 2 Corinthians 10: 3-5:

> "For though we live in the world, we do not
> wage war as the world does. The weapons we
> fight with are not the weapons of the world. On

the contrary, they have divine power to demolish strongholds. We demolish arguments and every pretension that sets itself up against the knowledge of God, and we take captive every thought to make it obedient to Christ."

Remember the strongholds we talked about? There was the jail made up of lies and deception. Lies and deception create walls in the mind that lock you up away from truth and freedom. Each lie works with the others to create a structure. The only way to demolish the structure (the jail) is to reject the lies and replace them with truth.

The Bible says we demolish arguments and take captive our thoughts to make them obedient to Christ. We demolish arguments and lies by comparing them with the truth we know from the word of God, the Bible, and from revelation given by the Holy Spirit.

Every lie and deception that is recognized must be repented of and pushed out of your mind by an act of your will. You must also choose to turn away from all attitudes and behaviors that are the result of believing the lie.

As truth is revealed and you take hold of it, you must part ways with all lies that the truth exposes. You must choose not to believe them any longer and must choose to believe the truth. This choice is not a feeling. Your emotions have been trained to respond to your thinking. As you part ways with old mindsets and beliefs your emotions are going to need some time to readjust to the new beliefs and truth you are receiving.

Take, for example, the man we talked about earlier who was told he was stupid and grew up thinking he was a failure. Suppose this man gets saved and begins the process of renewing his mind. The Holy Spirit starts pointing out to him the beliefs he has about himself that are wrong. He tells the man he is not stupid and not a failure. He tells him God made him wonderfully and that God has promised to cause him to be successful in what he does (Psalm 1). The man now has a choice to make. He must choose to believe what the Holy Spirit tells him instead of what his old programming tells him, and begin to act like he believes it. Every time the old, nagging thoughts of fear, rejection, and failure try to fill his mind, he must choose to push them out. He must not look to his emotions or feelings to tell him what is true, but to the word of God. As he does this, over time, the new beliefs begin to take hold and his emotions are re-trained to respond to the truth instead of lies.

This process is repeated for every lie and deception the Holy Spirit reveals. This is another reason why the renewal process takes time. For some people there are a lot of lies that have to be dealt with. Time must be allowed to come into agreement with truth and for belief in the truth to become a habit, just as formerly, believing the lie was a habit.

"My son, pay attention to what I say; listen closely to my words. Do not let them out of your sight, keep them within your heart; for they are life to those who find them and health to a man's whole body. Above all else, guard your heart, for it is the wellspring of life." (Proverbs 4: 20-23)

The heart here is synonymous with the mind. You are the keeper of your mind. You are the one who decides what gets to come in and what gets put out. No one else can do this for you. It is news to many people that they have a choice about what gets to come into their minds. Many have been passive for so long it's hard for them to break out of that mode and begin to pay attention to what they let themselves think about. At first it seems like a lot of work and takes a large amount of effort to police your thoughts. This is where you must be determined. It can seem overwhelming at first. This is only because you are not used to doing it.

You also have the ability to decide whether you will give in to your feelings or not. Our emotions are not to rule us; we are to rule them. This does not mean you deny what you feel. But you have the ability to decide whether or not you give in to your feelings or change them. You can choose to be cheerful even if you don't feel like it. You can choose to not allow negativity to rule you.

Prayer:

Father God, in Jesus' name, thank you for providing me with everything I need to renew my mind. Thank your for the Holy Spirit in me. Make me aware of thoughts and attitudes I entertain in my mind that need to be put out. I will resist these thoughts and attitudes and come out of agreement with them. I believe your grace is enough to give me the strength and wisdom to pull down every ungodly, untruthful structure in my mind.

I will no longer entertain these thoughts and attitudes but will push them out of my mind and cast them down. I will no longer give the devil a seat of authority and influence in my life by entertaining his lies and deceptions. I will rule over my mind by the grace of God and by the power of the Holy Spirit in me. Thank you for setting my mind free.

Dealing with the Jailers

As you are engaged in this process of giving up lies and choosing to believe truth, you may begin to notice the presence of jail guards you were not aware of before. Demons often guard the structures of lies we call strongholds and will resist attempts to tear them down. Often it is as a person begins to attempt to take control of their mind and thoughts that they become aware of the presence of demons that have been influencing their thinking and beliefs. They feel as if something is actively resisting them or fighting back as they attempt to change their thinking and rule over their minds. This brings us to the next step in the renewal process: dealing with any demonic forces that have gained access into your mind.

Demons are attached to lies and sin. Whatever lie or sin the demon is attached to must be repented of. There can be no entertaining of demons and their lies. All agreement with demonic thinking and beliefs must be broken and renounced. A demon of rejection (yes there is such a thing), for example, will attempt to enforce a rejection mindset. Thoughts and feelings of worthlessness, resentment, insecurity, fear of what others think, self-pity, failure, and defeat resulting from the demon's influence, must be firmly resisted. The demon will attempt to manipulate your emotions to reinforce ungodly, deceptive thinking. This, again is why you must not allow your emotions to determine what is true and what isn't.

All ungodly, untruthful thoughts associated with the demon must be cast down and pushed out of your mind. James says to resist the devil. This means you resist his influences and refuse to give in to them, whether they are influences to think or behave a certain way:

> "Submit yourselves, then, to God. Resist the devil, and he will flee from you." (James 4: 7)

I learned this one day when I went to the grocery store. As I was pushing the cart down the aisle I can only describe what I experienced as becoming extremely disoriented and feeling

124

overwhelming fear rise up in me that if I didn't leave the store right then I would freak out and lose it right there. It was my first experience with a really strong panic attack. I left my shopping cart right there in the aisle, walked out of the store, got in my car and started to drive home. As I was sitting at a left turn light waiting for it to turn green I started thinking.

I actually began to get kind of angry. When the light turned green, instead of going home, I went back to the store. I found my cart, still sitting in the aisle, and forced myself to finish my shopping. I went and stood in line to check out.

All during this time I could feel the things inside, trying to manifest and overwhelm me. I refused to give in to their influences. It was hard but I stood there in line until I finished paying for my stuff and then went home. It was a very important lesson. The demons couldn't make me do anything I didn't want to do and they had no power to take control of me and override my will. I found out I didn't have to let them have their way. I still needed to get them out, but I realized they could not just do whatever they wanted.

Whatever demons are present have to be identified and cast out. Some demonic oppression in the mind is the result of generational bondages that must be broken through repentance before the demon can be cast out. Curses related to occult sin, rebellion, sexual sin, and unforgiveness are some of the ones that can allow demonic powers to oppress and torment the mind.

To cast out the demons you address them by name (spirit of rejection, spirit of anger, spirit of deception, spirit of insanity etc.) and command them to leave in Jesus' name. You keep it up until evidence shows the demon has left. When the demon is gone, there will be a difference in the atmosphere of the mind. Unforgiveness, and sin that is not repented of will make

125

any attempts at deliverance useless.

Deliverance often comes by degrees rather than all at once. The person needs time to take control of each area of thinking and belief that was formerly bound up in lies and deception. Freedom comes as the truth is firmly established and the person is able to maintain control of their mind.

Pray and ask the Holy Spirit to open your eyes to the presence of any demons you need to deal with and to correctly identify them. Use your authority in Christ to command them to leave. Loose your mind from their control. Keep it up until you know they are gone. If you don't feel comfortable addressing them on your own, find someone who will pray with you and stand in faith with you for deliverance.

Demons I suspect might be influencing my mind:

_____

_____

_____

_____

_____

_____

Prayer:

Father God, thank you that you have given me authority to trample on snakes and scorpions and to overcome all the power of the enemy. Thank you for authority in the name of Jesus that demons must bow to. I exercise my kingdom authority against all demonic spirits that have infiltrated my mind and release myself from their control in Jesus name. All agreement between us is broken. You spirits of _____ (name the spirits), I command you to come out now in Jesus' name. Depart from me. I give you no more seat in my thinking and beliefs. I drive you out now by the Spirit of God and declare every yoke of bondage in my mind to be broken. Father, thank you for setting me free.

Filling up the tank

"Since, then, you have been raised with Christ, set your hearts on things above, where Christ is seated at the right hand of God. <u>Set your minds on things above, not on earthly things.</u>" (Colossians 3: 1-2)

"But we ought always to thank God for you, brothers and sisters loved by the Lord, because God chose you as firstfruits to be saved through the sanctifying work of the Spirit and <u>through belief in the truth.</u>" (2 Thessalonians 2: 13)

The last step we will discuss in renewing your mind is filling it with truth. A new structure of truth must be built to take the place of the old structure of lies that is being torn down. This is a mistake people sometimes make when dealing with renewing their mind. It is not enough to get rid of ungodly, untruthful thinking and beliefs. It is not enough to try to think positively. The jail that used to be in your mind must be replaced by a fortress built of truth. Your mind is not a vacuum. Something is going to fill it. It is not enough to stop believing lies. You must start believing and living out truth.

What I did to help fill my mind with truth was make a list of all the scriptures I could think of that talked to me about my situation, and dealt with the patterns of thinking that I needed to change. I wrote them all out on a piece of paper, not just the references. The list would grow as I found more scriptures and added them.

Every day I would take my list and read it out loud to myself sometimes up to two or three times a day. The warfare in my mind was so intense at times I needed constant reminders of truth. Hearing myself speaking the truth of the word (out loud) worked a change in me. I began to believe the things I was saying. Faith began to be built. The structures of the enemy were being demolished.

For each lie you listed earlier in this section, you are going to find a truth to replace it with. You will need a Bible and perhaps someone who can help show you where to look if you are not very familiar with what the Bible says. Find a scripture or scriptures that address the areas of your thinking that were once filled with lies. Write these scriptures down and begin to speak them out loud to yourself every day. An example of this would be replacing thoughts of resentment with choosing to forgive. Whenever old thoughts attempt to come back to your mind, push them out and begin to speak out the truth. This is called taking your medicine. If your doctor gave you medicine to take for an illness you would take it faithfully. God's word is medicine to your mind, restoring it to soundness and filling it with truth. Write your new truths below:

1. The truth about God:

_____

_____

_____

_____

_____

2. The truth about myself

_____

_____

_____

_____

3. The truth about other people

_____

_____

_____

_____

4. The truth about my life and circumstances.

_____

_____

_____

_____

_____

_____

The Bible is where you go to find truth and is the standard by which all revelation and input from other sources is judged as being truthful or not. It is the last word on truth and anything that departs from its truth must be rejected.

Our daily bread

"Man does not live on bread alone, but on every word that comes from the mouth of God." (Matthew 4: 4)

Every day you need to eat so your body can function properly. Your inner person must be fed daily too. Constantly having the truth in the front of your mind keeps you from forgetting it. The enemy's lies can often be so smooth and convincing that if you don't keep the truth in front of you all the time you can be deceived.

Adam and Eve were in a perfect place where there was no sin and they didn't have to deal with a world that was under the control of the devil. That didn't keep Eve from being deceived. We must remember we are still living in a fallen world that is without the true knowledge of God and every day we are bombarded with thoughts, feelings, ideas etc. from this world. We must choose to fill our minds continually with truth:

"Finally, brothers, whatever is true (notice what is first on the list!), whatever is noble, whatever is right, whatever is pure, whatever is lovely, whatever is admirable – if anything is excellent or praiseworthy – think about such things." (Philippians 4: 8)

Remember, you choose what you allow into your mind. Here Paul is saying you must guard your mind and be careful about what you entertain there. If your mind is filled with truth, deception will not be able to get in. In your fortress of truth you will be protected from the weapons and flaming darts of the devil. All of the lies you used to believe must be replaced with truth. If you are not sure what the truth is, find out.

For example, if you have struggled with rejection you could go to the Bible and read in Ephesians:

"For he chose us in him before the creation of the world to be holy and blameless in his sight. In love he predestined us to be adopted as his sons through Jesus Christ, in accordance with his pleasure and will . . ."(Ephesians 1: 4-5)

"But because of his great love for us, God, who is rich in mercy, made us alive with Christ even when we were dead in transgressions . . ." (Ephesians 2: 4)

"Consequently you are no longer foreigners and aliens, but fellow citizens with God's people and members of God's household . . ." (Ephesians 2: 19)

Here you have presented the truth of how God feels about you, how much he loves you. Knowing this truth presents you with a choice. You can continue to choose to believe you are unloved and unwanted or you can choose to believe what the word says, that you are God's child, greatly loved, and therefore accepted and secure.

The fortress of truth is built whenever you make the choice to believe the truth and reject the lie. It is your responsibility to search out the truth and begin to renew your mind. The best way to fill your mind with truth is to make sure you spend enough time in the Bible every day to become familiar with it. Reading the word, studying it, hearing it preached and taught by others, praying it, speaking it out loud, and singing it (making up songs using the scriptures for the words) are all ways you can keep the truth in the forefront of your mind.

Another way to fill yourself with truth is to pray in the Spirit in your heavenly prayer language. (If you are not baptized in the Holy Spirit, read Acts 2) The Spirit of Truth dwells in you and when you speak in tongues you are giving voice to the truth as the Spirit prays through you (1 Corinthians 14:4-5a; 15). As you pray in the Spirit your natural mind is illuminated; revelation, wisdom, and understanding are released to you:

> "Do not get drunk on wine, which leads to debauchery. Instead, be filled with the Spirit. Speak to one another with psalms, hymns and spiritual songs. Sing and make melody in your heart to the Lord, always giving thanks to God the Father for everything, in the name of our Lord Jesus Christ." (Ephesians 5: 18-19)

> "Let the word of Christ dwell in you richly as you teach and admonish one another with all wisdom, and as you sing psalms, hymns and spiritual songs with gratitude in your hearts to

God." (Colossians 3: 16)

Below, write your plan of action for how you will fill your mind up with truth. Make it something that you will actually be able to do. Don't say you will read your Bible for 5 hours a day if you know you won't be able to keep that commitment. At the same time, challenge yourself a little bit. Reading 1 or 2 verses a day will probably not fill you up very quickly. It takes a long time to eat bread if you only eat one crumb at a time.

Pray and ask God to show you what the best method is for you. Include the things we talked about earlier: reading the word, studying, attending services where the word will be taught and you can be encouraged, etc. You can also try to find someone who will be able to mentor you and help you with this process:

My plan of action:

_____

_____

_____

_____

_____

_____

_____

_____

14

The Prophetic - God's Truth About You

> "But the one who prophesies speaks to people for their strengthening, encouraging and comfort." (1 Corinthians 14:3)

There is probably nothing that has more power to change your thinking and beliefs than a word spoken to you by the inspiration of the Spirit. When you receive a word of exhortation, edification, or comfort from someone by the Spirit of God, truth is imparted to you in a very powerful way.

A prophetic word is God's truth about you and your life. It is a glimpse into the way he sees you and into what he created you to be. This is why prophetic ministry is so important. This is why Paul told the Corinthian believers, "Follow the way of love and eagerly desire gifts of the Spirit, especially prophecy" (1 Corinthians 14:1). The words "eagerly desire" have the connotation of actually lusting after something.

A word of prophecy can cut through deception like a knife. Maybe that's why the devil tries so hard to shut it down. The Corinthian church was full of people who needed to have their minds renewed. Paul exhorted them to become proficient in the gift of prophecy.

You have to remember in those days there were no printed Bibles that everyone had access to. I believe Paul was encouraging the Corinthian church to develop their spiritual gifts, especially prophecy as a way for them to receive revelation from the Holy Spirit that would help them renew their minds and change their thinking.

Many of us have received prophetic words from different people as part of our Christian experience. God gives them to us for a reason. They are part of the campaign of the Holy Spirit to renew our minds and tear down strongholds of ungodly thinking. A word of prophecy will act as an anchor to keep us grounded in truth and as a compass to direct our steps as we make choices and decisions every day:

> "Timothy, my son, I am giving you this command in keeping with the prophecies once made about you, so that by recalling them (the prophecies) you may fight the battle well, holding on to faith and a good conscience, which some have rejected and so have suffered shipwreck with regard to the faith." (1 Timothy 1: 18-19)

Paul is telling Timothy to let the prophetic words he has received be his guide to direct his steps. These prophetic words are God's truth about Timothy. They are his guide to tell him what to think about himself and his purpose, what choices he needs to make to fulfill his purpose, and to keep him centered in that place. They help him see the thoughts, lies, deception, and distractions from the enemy that he needs to put away and separate himself from.

Living, active words

Prophecy is an important part of renewing your mind and cleaning your filter out. Through prophetic ministry, you receive truth about yourself, about God, about other people, and about your circumstances and life. A prophetic word can enable you to steer a clear course through the maze of life and to see yourself as God sees you. As you receive and come into agreement with the truth that is imparted through prophecy your thinking and mindsets adjust to conform to that truth. There is nothing like an accurate prophetic word to totally change your perspective and thinking. That is why we are told:

> "Do not treat prophecies with contempt but test them all; hold on to what is good, reject every kind of evil . . ." (1 Thessalonians 5: 20)

All prophecy needs to be tested and judged. Many Christians don't pay much attention to prophecy because they have had a bad experience with someone who spoke to them in the name of the Lord and led them astray. This doesn't need to happen. It is your job to test the words people give you.

Even when the Corinthians were messing up with regard to how they used the spiritual gifts, Paul's answer was not to tell them to stop prophesying but to learn how to do it right. We must judge prophecies by the written word, the Bible, by comparing them to other prophecies we have received, and by the witness of the Holy Spirit inside us, as to whether or not they are really from God. A few words that were not really spoken by the Spirit of God do not nullify all the ones that were. Learning to discern the source of prophecy sharpens your perception and teaches you to tell the difference between truth and lies.

Your prophetic words will give you a picture of your God-given identity and purpose. They will show you what God has deposited in you that he wants to cause to grow and come to maturity. They will help you see any lies and deception that may be part of your thinking. Your prophetic words are a road map to direct you into the place and purpose God has for you to function in his kingdom. They tell you the truth about yourself. You have the choice to believe and come into agreement with this truth or ignore it or reject it.

Take a moment right now to think about any prophecies that you have received. If you have them written down or recorded somewhere it would be a good idea to go read them or listen to them again. Allow the Holy Spirit to remind you of the truth about yourself and your life. Ask him to show you any mindsets or beliefs you may have that are not in agreement with what has been spoken into your life.

Prayer:

Heavenly Father,

Thank you that your eye is on me continually; that the thoughts you have concerning me are more than the sand of the sea. Thank you for the prophetic words that have been given to me. In Jesus' name, help me take hold of the truths I have received through these words. Show me any place where I am allowing ungodly, untruthful thinking or mindsets to keep me from embracing these truths. I choose to believe what you have said concerning me, my life, and purpose. I reject and renounce everything that does not agree with what you have said about me. I choose to let these prophetic words guide my thinking and beliefs about me and my life. I will let them be my road map and compass and will fight the good fight to take hold of what you have said to me. Renew my mind in truth so I can walk in the light instead of the dark. In Jesus' name, Amen

Write down here the picture God has given, through the prophetic words you have received, of who you are and what your God-given purpose and destiny are:

_____

_____

_____

_____

_____

_____

_____

Perhaps you have never received a word of prophecy. Ask the Holy Spirit to give you revelation so you can see yourself as God sees you and so you can see what he has created you to be and to do. This revelation may come through a dream or vision, or it may come through a person God will send into your life.

Whatever way it comes, you can be sure that God wants to speak to you about the plans he has for you. He wants to show you what you look like from his point of view (don't worry, it's good!). God sees your end from the beginning. He wants to show you what you need to see so you can walk together with him in love, fellowship, and purpose.

Prayer:

Heavenly Father,

Show me who I am in Jesus; who and what you have created me to be. Show me the pieces that make up the picture of my life. I want to hear from you. I want to know the thoughts you have concerning me. I need you to give me the roadmap and compass that will keep me on the straight and narrow road. I want your involvement in my life to be up close and personal! Give me a dream. Send someone to give me the word you have for me so my mind can be renewed in truth. I will wait in expectation to hear what you have to say. Thank you.

In Jesus' name,

Amen

Epilogue

The Last Word

I hope this book has been helpful to you. There is such a need for God's people to have their minds renewed so they can come into agreement with God's plans and purposes and stop living confused, aimless lives. Renewing the mind is a process, not a one-time event. It takes place over time. But every step you take along the way brings you closer to walking with God every day in true fellowship and love. Seeing the world and your life from his eternal perspective is a wonderful thing. Everything falls into place when you know the truth and commit to living according to it.

Don't be discouraged if you feel like you have a lot of stuff to deal with. If God could get me through he can get you through too. God already knows about it all and has everything worked out for getting you to where you need to go. His timetable for you is just right. Don't fall into the trap of trying to compare yourself with other people. Trust God to work in you exactly what you need.

If you have been helped by reading this, find someone who is struggling and see if you can help them find the way out of their own jail. Going from the place of needing help to being able to give help can do wonders for your thinking and perception! Let's work together so the entire body of Christ will be whole and healthy and so the world will get a truthful picture of God's kingdom people. Blessings.

Notes:

Notes: